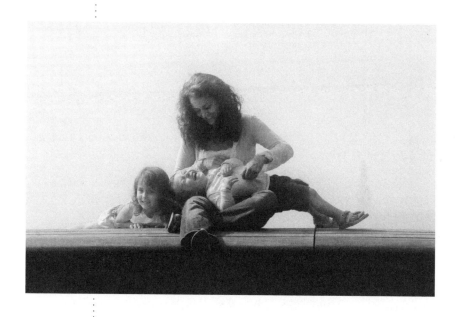

For my children with all my love always
Love yourselves and each other with your whole heart

Savannah
Born under the Stars and the Moon
Creative and Beautiful
September 18, 2000, 5:19 a.m.

&

Orion
Born with the rising Sun
Joyful and Powerful
April 27, 2003, 8:13 a.m.

Better Birth

The Ultimate Guide to Childbirth from Home Births to Hospitals

Denise Spatafora
Creator of the BornClear Method

WILEY
John Wiley & Sons, Inc.

Copyright © 2009 by Denise Spatafora. All rights reserved

Published by John Wiley & Sons, Inc., Hoboken, New Jersey
Published simultaneously in Canada

Photograph on p. iii by Stefanie Jasper. All other photographs are courtesy of Timothi Jane Graham.

For general information about our other products and services, please contact our Customer Care Department within the United States at (800) 762-2974, outside the United States at (317) 572-3993 or fax (317) 572-4002.

Wiley also publishes its books in a variety of electronic formats. Some content that appears in print may not be available in electronic books. For more information about Wiley products, visit our web site at www.wiley.com.

Library of Congress Cataloging-in-Publication Data:

Spatafora, Denise.
   Better birth: the ultimate guide to childbirth from home births to hospitals/
Denise Spatafora.
      p.   cm.
   Includes index.
      ISBN 978-0-470-25561-2 (pbk.)
      1. Childbirth—Popular works.   2. Childbirth at home—Popular works.   I. Title.
RG525.S647   2009
618.4—dc22

                                                                              2008055887

Printed in the United States of America

10 9 8 7 6 5 4 3 2 1

Contents

Foreword

By Candace B. Pert, Ph.D, Chief Scientific Officer,
RAPID Pharmaceuticals, Rockville, Maryland

Finally, someone has taken the science of the mind-body connection and applied it to the experience of childbirth. The era of medical birth primacy and its treatment of women as bodies without mind, emotion, or spirit, is over.

Thanks to Denise Spatafora, a new era of smart birth—women and their partners being fully empowered to design birthing experiences of their choice—is upon us. Denise is a woman with a mission, and with BornClear she launches a movement to alter forever how we approach and conduct ourselves through conception, pregnancy, birthing, and parenting. She is up to no less than a revolution in consciousness.

Knowledge is access, and the access Denise is offering through BornClear is grounded in the scientific discoveries I and my colleagues made in the 1970s while I was first at Johns Hopkins and later at the National Institutes of Mental Health in Bethesda, Maryland. As described in my book *Molecules of Emotion*, I laid the foundation for the discovery of endorphin, the body's natural morphine and the brain chemical responsible for the exhilarating emotion of bliss and pain-free childbirth, among other effects. That groundbreaking research led to the even more astounding finding in the 1980s that each of us is a communication network of chemical information. The mind and the body are constantly in communication, a process that is highly regulated by the molecules of emotion, the peptides, of which the endorphin is one.

In the work I did with my team to establish the mind-body connection, I showed how conscious breathing, a technique employed by both the yogi during meditation and the woman in labor, can alter the experience of pain. There is a wealth of data showing that changes in the rate and the depth of breathing produce changes in the quantity and the kind of chemicals that are released from the brain—and vice versa. You can cause those chemicals, by consciously controlling your breath—a principle used in Lamaze and other birthing techniques — to diffuse rapidly throughout the cerebrospinal fluid and thus diminish your pain. The endorphin-respiratory link is well documented. Virtually any endorphin molecule found anywhere else can be found in the respiratory center, providing the scientific rationale for the powerful healing effects of consciously controlled breath patterns.

My science led me to trust my body as I went through becoming pregnant and giving birth to my own children. After one high-tech, heavily drugged hospital delivery and a second natural childbirth, again in the environment of a hospital, I'd decided to have my third child at home. At that time, I continued to be my own best laboratory rat, experimenting on myself to prove or disprove my theses. I wanted to be emotionally present for the birth and fully in control of the process.

I knew about the breathing connection to endorphin release, and so I used conscious controlled breathing, a surefire, proven strategy for releasing endorphins and quelling pain, to experience a natural, pain-diminished delivery of my child. I trusted my instincts and the wisdom of my body, something I'd been prevented from doing in the hospital environment, with its emphasis on high-tech machinery over mind-body wisdom. It was an experience that won me over to natural childbirth.

Another aspect I love about the BornClear approach is Denise's understanding of how knowledge dispels fear. In this book, Denise arms women and their partners with an incredible amount of knowledge—not only about the development of the fetus, as so many books do, but about the relationship of our thoughts, feelings, and beliefs to the experiences of being pregnant, giving birth, and parenting.

My work has shown that we all filter our perceptions of reality through a network of emotional chemicals, highly coloring what we see as "out there," or objective reality. The quality and freedom of those emotions—whether they are stuck and suppressed or flowing and alive—can profoundly impact that experience. Preparing for childbirth and parenting has everything to do with our thoughts and feelings, and knowing this can give you an advantage in having a beautiful, joyful experience, rather than a frightening and painful one.

Denise has walked her talk—she is a mother like myself and has used her own experience of birthing two children to empower others and further her own personal growth and evolution. She has supported countless women and their partners, children, and families to choose freely, armed with the latest knowledge science has to offer. In BornClear, she makes her vast experience available, and for that we can all be thankful.

Acknowledgments

As I think, a few days before my own birthday, about all the amazing people who have contributed to this book and to my life, I am moved by how much love and gratitude I feel. Feeling known, appreciated, and acknowledged are some of the greatest gifts you can give a human being, so I hope you all know that I see you, appreciate you, and will always be thankful for you.

First, my family. Thank you, Mom (Irene), for giving birth to me and for the depth of your love and support. I am grateful for your showing me a magic that I was able to turn into a language. You know me. You are beautiful in every way, and I love you more than words can express. Richard, my stepfather, you are such a special man and grandfather and you have graced our lives. I love you. To my sister, Cinzia, to whom I am so deeply connected, I know we will always be there for each other. I deeply love you and your spirit. Much love to my brother-in-law, Bennett, and my nieces and nephew, Alexandria, Charlotte, and Chase—we are family at the core. Thank you, Uncle Eugene, for being there for me in bright and dark moments with your joy and reassurance. You are my guardian angel. To my father, Anthony, with much peace and love—thank you.

Savannah and Orion, my children, to whom I have dedicated this book with all my heart, and my partner, David Raine. David—of course you know I am crying as I write this—you are my love and my king. I am your queen, and you help me feel like one every day. I asked the universe for a man who was spiritually and emotionally intelligent, a beautiful artist who was true to himself, willing to fearlessly create life, a partner in making a difference in the world, a playmate; that man is you. Thank you for seeing and loving me. Thank you for teaching me the power and beauty of joy, for all the beautiful songs you have written, for loving and teaching Savannah and Orion in the way that you do—relentlessly present and with humor, God's music. Thank you for the best blessings at dinnertime. You always know the right words to capture all of the dimensions of whatever is happening—so clear and knowing. Thank you for writing the last paragraph of this book—perfect! We are partners. I know you and love you. Hallelujah anyhow!

Much love and hugs to Horus, our family dog, the god of perception, and our celebrated character actor.

To my extended family, aunts, uncles, grandparents, cousins, nieces, and nephews in the Spatafora, Belsito, and Salerno families—much love and blessings. I am grateful for our rich, wise, and complex lineage.

For the initiation of this book, thank you to my agent, Carol Mann, who is always confident and clear.

To my co-writer, Pam Liflander, thank you for your partnership, for relentlessly working with me, for your groundedness, for your sense of humor, and for ensuring the clarity of my voice—it has been a divine and important process and I am forever grateful. To Christel Winkler from John Wiley & Sons—thank you for seeing my vision and knowing the difference we all wanted to make from the moment we began working together.

The experts and contributors to this book generously provided wisdom and knowledge that are both overwhelming and beautiful. I thank them with all the gratitude I can summon for helping me to fulfill the BornClear mission to make a profound difference for millions of people and newborn babies: Dr. Eden Fromberg; Dr. Candice Pert; Cara Muhlhahn; Dr. Marsden Wagner; Ina May Gaskin; Dr. Joe Dispenza; Barbara Powers; Dr. David Chamberlain; Angela Le; all of the amazing yoga teachers including Elena Brower and Nikki Costello of Virayoga,

Latham Thomas of Tender Shoots Wellness, and Deb Flashenberg of the Prenatal Yoga Center, New York City; Mia Borgatta of Lilawellness; Patricia Moreno; Dr. Jacques Moritz; Patricia Schermerhorn; Nancy Marriott; Dr. Michel Odent; Armando Morones; Dr. Michel Cohen; Barbara Harper; Meg Richichi, Julia Indichova, Heather Arak, and Nathan Kanofsky; Daphne Beal, Angie Clarke, Brett Hoebel, Andi Silverman, Annemarie Colbin, Ina Bransome, and Haya Brant; Ali Wing; Soho Parenting; DONA; Tania Ketenjian and Ahri Golden; Agnes Chapski; Karen Gurwitz, and all of the BornClear resources throughout the United States featured in this book and on the BornClear Web site.

Thank you to all of my friends, my clients, my angels, my tribe, and my soul sisters: Raja Shaheen, godmother, high priestess; Marla Supnick, wisdom, love; Eli Kuslansky, playmate, mystic; Ava, loving, creative; Gloria Bermudiz, knowing, courageous; Venessa Giordano, playful, questions; Kathryn Jaliman, grace, divinity; Pam Wolf, inspiring, fun; Melanie Englese, passionate, loyal; Lisa Chiccine, beauty, warmth; Jill Mangino, magical, generous; Roberta Scott, my midwife (My journey all started with you. Love you); Bonnie Kramen, smile, expansive; Justine Lackey, mystical, synchronicity; Lauren Zander, earth angel, sister; David Zander, music, loving; Beth Weissenberger, clear, loving; Armin Weissenberger, committed, anchor; Maryann Gonzales, peaceful, special; Linda Falzarano, *Oh Namah Shivaya*, beautiful; Lisa Bernstein, willing, humble; Nicole Heidbreder, earth mother, healing; Kelly Duignan, divine, fluid; Dan Shaw, wise, good; Lisa Robbins, beauty, synchronicity; Heath Robbins, creative, powerful; Ken Robbins, thank you; Judy Robbins, inspiration, feminine; Hayley Sue Babcock, special, loving; Shannon Spellman, teacher, adventurous; Kevin Hart, organic, artist; Emmanuel Faccio, laughter, passion; Adri Trigiani, saint, wise; Maggie Shapiro, loving, loyal, wise; Lucy Rector Fillppo, funny, self-expressed; Timothi Jane Graham, goddess, free; Pamela Morgan, passionate, curious; the Feltes family, loving, willing; Lynn San Andres, joyful, faith; Nelle Fortenberry, compassion, creativity; Connie Connors, the wind, pinky promise; Heather Lord, stillness, poetry; Tami Zaroff, patience, *Sadguru na maharaj ki jay*; Mary Margrill, green apple, loving; Jenn Contini and Leo, family, pasta; Lesley Provenzano, beautiful, generous; Holly

Strutt, artist, generous; Macarena, smile, mommy; Amy Beth Sestito, trust, pleasure; Kate Rolston, special, world traveler; Geraldine Agren, seer, soul; Ellie Gordon, boundless, Earth; Maria Napoli, airbender, channel; Ruth Thomas, courageous, contribution; Lisa Zimmerman, kind, signs; Laurie Kuslansky, intimate, powerfully vulnerable; Heidi Krupp, joyous, believe; Leslie Stevens, friend, limitless; Martha McCully, artist, loving; Regina Kulik Scott, courageous, trailblazer; Jane Shamanesh, open, big; Nicole Gabai, kind, tender; James Smith, clarity, trust; Graceann Bennett, fluid, fun; Marcia Nelson, so loving, connected; Jasmine Djerradine, beautiful Libra, clear.

Jacqueline Beaudette, same tribe, familiar; Karen O'Brian, clear, wise; Ariel Villafane and the beautiful group of women, divine, safe; Lynn Kreaden, loving, galaxy traveler; Kate Baum, certainty, steadfastness; Robert Singerman, creative, generous; Mathew and Louise Evins, I just love you; Stephanie Campbell, change, excitement; Regina Conceicao, special, divine lineage; Ross Rayburn, willing, heart; Lucio Zago, Sicily, ease; Patricia Saraceni, beauty, *amicizia*; Cathy O'Brian, warm, worldly; Maryann Zoellner, the beginning of the sign to do this book; Susan Osborne, supportive, acknowledging; Erica Bartman, courageous, ready; Holly Hatfield of the Chopra Center, New York City, thank you! To Shaun T. of "Insanity" and all the staff and participants, thank you. You helped me become so strong, physically as well as mentally, supporting me in "walking my talk."

My Dorset, Vermont, community: Pam Reed, brilliant, knowing; Marsha Norman, tickle backs, sharing; Kit and Dan Mosheim, infinite love and generosity; Fran Sirak, knowing eyes; Ted Parisi, Sicilian, protector; Marion McChesney, generous and earthy; Gregor, entertaining and delicious; Melanie of Chantecleer, always warm; Laura Beckwith, intuition, trust; Lisa Chalidze, freedom fighter, laughter; Elizabeth Torak, language with paint, goddess; and Lisa Helmholz Adams, honesty, power, soul.

The loving amazing communities that have been like family around my children from day one, including Sarah and Becky Bovey of Rabbit Hill Preschool in Dorset, Vermont—a sacred, fun, enchanted community for Savannah that also included Amy and Lily Thebault, Fred and Rusty—thank you so much for everything.

Clara and Bob Basalari, Orion's godparents and true angels, who supported me in raising Orion during his first few years with such love and devotion, I am forever grateful. Julie Staub, our babysitter for two years—thank you for your endless love, commitment, and, of course, the unforgettable photographs. All of our friends, families, and teachers at our schools, which include the Montessori School of Manhattan, Claremont Preparatory School, and our current school PS89 here in Tribeca, New York City; Rachel Goldstein and Joy Marchese and all of the volunteers at Spirituality for Kids; and the Downtown Soccer League Community, New York City. I am so grateful for our piano teacher of many years, Leslie Upchurch. Our babysitter, Carly Clarke—so loving and playful. We are so happy you are in our lives. To the many amazing women and their partners, who have taken the BornClear course over the years, including Steve and Deb Grant, Belinda Clarke, Liz Willette, Elisa and Larry Rader, Laurie Gerber and Will Craig, Jill Ordonez, Diedre Decaro, Catie Riggs, Claire Wallington, Elena Caffentzis, Angelica Feigin, Paola Weintraub and Nick Gomez, Danielle Spaeth, Nicole Adams, Den Bradley, Karen and Dori Gurwitz—thank you for your trust and the journeys you took. To all my coaching/consulting clients and companies over the years, including Neal Goldman and Peter Kellner, Gray Hudkins, Glenn Laumeister, Graceann Bennett, Joshua Cooper Ramo, Daniel Dubno, Daphne Kis, Jay Lauf, Peggy Traub, Sammy Sitt, Claudine Loi, Susan and Peter Laughter, and Ali and Betty Riaz—thank you for all we created together and for being the trailblazers that you are.

To all those I have not mentioned who have touched me, taught me, and inspired me, your impact allowed me to pass the inspiration on to others. Please know who you are. And thank you!

Just as leaves lie quietly until a strong wind whips them into an inspired frenzy of whispering and wise secret sharing, so does our emotional, moving energy whip us into a frenzy of loving and joy sharing. When the leaves gently touch Earth, sometimes miles from their last landing, they have seen and shared countless wise secrets.

I too have made this commitment to my way of life. I will forever allow myself to whip into wonderful, passionate frenzies, all the while seeing, then sharing.

Introduction

The way we have come to expect a "traditional" pregnancy and birthing to look and feel has dramatically changed in our modern, technically enhanced times. The once customary rite of passage, with its inherent understanding that women were designed to give birth, has morphed into a sterile and oftentimes lonely medical procedure. This shift in thinking has inadvertently led us into an era where many women feel as if they are bringing new life into this world without really being present for the experience.

Before the 1920s, most births took place at home and were attended by doctors or midwives, but by the 1930s women were flocking to hospitals, hoping to experience the revolutionary methods of "painless" childbirth. Even though the doctors of the time did not deliver on this ridiculous promise, we continued to follow and "improve" on these

1

new scientific practices, and before we knew it, we had unintentionally relinquished control over the entire childbirth experience. Every aspect of hospitalized childbirth became almost mechanical, and they were all orchestrated by a doctor. Women were separated from their husbands, sedated by drugs that made them oblivious to the birthing process, and kept in sterile environments. Breast-feeding was discouraged, and breast milk was replaced by "enhanced" infant formulas. As time passed, we completely forgot how to own and control pregnancy and childbirth: the natural, normal aspects of delivery no longer existed.

Doctors gave great arguments to pregnant mothers. As Dr. David Chamberlain, an expert in prenatal psychology, said, "The doctor's byline was, 'Let us do it. Trust me; we know how to do this.' But they didn't. All they had to offer was a protocol. They treated every mother the same, every father the same and every baby the same."

According to the World Health Organization, "By medicalizing birth, i.e., separating woman from her own environment and surrounding her with strange people using strange machines to do strange things to her in an effort to assist her, the woman's state of mind and body is so altered that her way of carrying through this intimate act must also be altered and the state of the baby born must equally be altered. The result is that it is no longer possible to know what births would have been like before these manipulations—they have no idea what 'non-medicalized' birth is. The entire modern obstetric . . . literature is essentially based on observations of 'medicalized' birth."

Before women could muster up opinions to the contrary, technology took hold once again, to the point where today the Cesarean section is the most common form of surgery performed in any hospital. According to the National Center for Health Statistics, 1 in 3 babies in the United States is delivered by Cesarean section. *USA Today* reported that in 2006, 31.1 percent of U.S. births were by C-section, a 50 percent increase over the previous decade. Some doctors are even referring to C-sections as *vaginal bypass surgery*! While C-sections can be lifesaving operations when either the mother or the baby faces certain health-related problems, many health-care experts believe that a good number of C-sections are performed unnecessarily. Too often, they are scheduled to meet the personal needs of obstetricians or the hospital staff or to conform to the hectic lives of mothers themselves.

In almost every country in the world outside of the United States, 75 to 80 percent of all low-risk pregnancies are attended by midwives. In the United States, most women are still opting for a hospital birth, but many report afterward that their experiences were less than ideal and sometimes traumatic. Often, they are disappointed with the clinical character of the process. Women often say that they felt as if they were not included in their childbirth. Other mothers have told me that even though they were well informed about "what to expect," they were too scared of the pain to be emotionally present, so they relinquished control to the medical team. They did not know how to deal with the totality of the experience in real time because they really weren't prepared.

On top of individual experiences, the main conversation about birthing that is often shared among traditional health-care providers, birthing professionals, and even girlfriends is that childbirth is a painful ordeal, an uncomfortable means to an end. The discussion then compartmentalizes the process into two categories: "successful" mainstream or "alternative" vaginal births, and "unfortunate" or "scheduled" C-sections.

Yet this negative and limiting conversation doesn't have to exist at all. Today, many women, as well as mainstream health-care professionals, are speaking up against the current culture of childbirth, and changes are happening, even in hospitals. Doctors and midwives are uniting to find better solutions to the increasing rate of C-sections, as well as the rising costs of hospital births. Husbands and partners have reentered the birthing room. Mothers are encouraged to breast-feed by both ob-gyns and pediatricians: medical statistics now back up what many women have known all along, that breast-feeding is the healthiest feeding option for both mother and baby.

The next step is for pregnant women to relearn the true experience of childbirth. We deserve to have a say in the medications we take or decide not to take. We need options so that we can decide where we will deliver our babies and who will be present at the delivery. We can take personal responsibility in creating exactly the kind of the childbirth we want. We want to be treated as partners instead of as patients. We want to bond with our children immediately after their birth. And we want to design and create a childbirth that is safe, peaceful, and secure. These ideals are what BornClear is all about.

The absolute truth is that there are no rules when it comes to creating what you really want for your childbirth and for every aspect of your life. In fact, there aren't any rules except the ones you make up. The BornClear program was created out of my own experiences. When I was first pregnant, I searched for new as well as ancient ways to create a peaceful and memorable birth. I wanted to fully educate myself, so I pulled information from many resources, piecing together and creating exactly what I needed to be mentally, emotionally, and physically ready. I started to prepare my body for birth by learning to control the connection between my mind and my body through a variety of mental and physical practices that included prenatal yoga, meditation, and deep relaxation. Over the course of my journey, I became able to fully trust my natural birthing instincts, as well as my body, and I found myself tapping into a deeper, more enlightened space in my mind.

Nine months later, I witnessed the birth of my daughter. What impressed me most was that I felt completely awake and present to the divinity and wonder of the birth. Two years later, I experienced the same with my son, whose birth was also peaceful and beautiful. My life's work has always been about teaching others how to create lives they can be proud of. After my childbirth experiences, I decided to focus this mission more specifically to be able to share my extensive birthing knowledge and life practice tools with other women.

The BornClear approach that I have developed works whether you plan on giving birth at a hospital, at a birthing center, or at home. What's most important is being mentally, physically, and spiritually prepared so that you can create the birthing experience you want for yourself and your family.

As a business and life coach I have worked with private individuals and public companies, including Google, Condé Nast, Citibank, Ogilvy & Mather, Dove (Unilever), BBC, Credit Suisse, and others. I have coached CEOs, their teams, entrepreneurs, athletes, celebrities, and hundreds of people just like you. My gift is that I can feel, hear, and see all that is limiting a person and/or a business as well as their gifts. As their coach, I make my agenda their agenda—which is to uncover and actualize their commitment and dreams. I find that

I can make the biggest difference when people are willing to look at how their thoughts, beliefs, behaviors, and habits affect their own satisfaction, their lives, and the impact they have on others and the world. I have had the great fortune that my clients have trusted me to help them self-correct, release their fears, and be free to be successful in whatever they are pursuing.

The BornClear course is an extension of this same practice. I started teaching it in 2001 and have been building its success ever since. The classes run every few weeks, and I am creating a nationwide teacher training program, as well as developing a DVD of the course.

BornClear is a one-day program that we teach to a group of ten to fifteen couples. We also provide individual follow-up from the time each couple begins the course until the birth of their child. The class is designed to be completed in one day in order to fit into most people's busy schedules. More important, the curriculum builds on itself, steeping the couples fully in the "space" of birth. This book includes all of the elements that are covered in the course.

I find that whether I'm working with couples or expectant mothers, people limit themselves when they don't take the time to understand their inner selves, including their reactions to the intrinsic fears that prevent them from tapping in to their own power. All of the elements and the dimensions I deal with in my coaching/consulting practice and all of the philosophies and practices I developed in regard to understanding human beings and behavior, plus my own life lessons and experiences, have been integrated into designing and leading the BornClear course and writing this book.

It is always deeply inspiring to watch the couples in the workshop transform. Very often, they start one way—resistant, afraid, confused, disconnected—and end in another: in a place of clarity, empowerment, and deep connection with their dreams, their commitments, and each other. Even after they complete the course, I love to hear from participants how BornClear changed their lives—how it even helped them address issues outside of their birthing experience. It is moving and beautiful when people get to the heart of themselves, where they can discover what really matters to them and their new family. Starting a family—beginning a child's life—from this place is my gift to these couples, and I am always moved by the knowledge that the "babies" in the course are learning and experiencing too.

The BornClear Program

The mission of my class and of this book has both individual and global goals. First, this book aims to give you all of the tools—including my extensive knowledge and my best practices—that will help you address and resolve your unique physical, mental, emotional, and spiritual concerns regarding conception and childbirth. This book has been designed to be a comprehensive resource that encompasses everything you will need to be fully prepared.

There are seven basic lessons in the BornClear program. By following the program, you will:

- Understand the power of the mind-body connection and how it relates to every aspect of pregnancy, from conception all the way through childbirth. The mind-body connection actually encourages the body's ability to produce the natural chemicals that can modulate how we experience the sensations of pregnancy and childbirth. These chemicals are an important aspect of controlling how fast labor comes and how comfortable we are during labor. You will come to understand how your thoughts can affect your pregnancy and birth, on both an emotional and a physical level.

- Determine early in your pregnancy what you deeply desire for your own birthing experience. You will learn how to become more introspective and tap into what you really want and need to fulfill your choices. In order to do this, you will learn how to explore your own fears, concerns, and worries. Once you have managed these issues, you will be able to move past your concerns and become completely at ease with your pregnancy, now and going forward.

- Have the necessary tools to call on during conception, pregnancy, and birth. I call this the BornClear toolbox. Included are original breathing techniques, meditations, visualizations, and other mental and physical exercises that I have developed and successfully used with my clients.

- Connect and align with your baby during pregnancy to create emotional, spiritual, and health bonds that will last a lifetime.

- Fully understand how your body works during pregnancy and childbirth. You will learn how to create a more comfortable birth by deepening your mind-body connection and learning to control your attitudes and thoughts, as well as your physical body. In this way, you will be fully prepared for each stage of labor.

- Have the ability to plan ahead for every contingency. Careful preparation and planning ensure that each parent is clear about the details of childbirth. You will learn how to create and initiate the right conversations, including questions you will need to ask your birth team (doctor/midwife/doula). You will also discover how to create alignment with your partner and how to make plans for the future after the baby is born.

- Begin to envision the first year after birth by learning your options in many realms, including breast-feeding, circumcision, and more. Most important, you will discover how to take care of yourself, your partner, and your baby.

Birthing a New Beginning

Underlying all of the preparations for this pregnancy and childbirth is a second goal: that you will grow personally. You can use this program to become more emotionally fulfilled as you learn how to trust and honor yourself. Once you have completed the exercises and learned the lessons in this book, you will be fully prepared for the challenges that lie ahead, not only when you deliver your new baby, but as you approach your new life as a parent.

This gift of self-awareness is also crucial in having a comfortable childbirth, but it is the one component that women often neglect. Without it, we have been forced to surrender fertility issues and the birthing of our children to a script defined by someone else, be it a doctor, a nurse, a midwife, friends, or even the media. This is why many women describe childbirth merely as the few hours they spent in a delivery room, instead of focusing on the lessons they learned during the entire pregnancy.

My main goal is to globally change the way we perceive and talk about childbirth. I want to empower all women so that childbirth is no longer talked about as "surviving an ordeal." For this to happen, women have to take control of this experience. That is why I want every woman to be able to harness this gift—the ability to trust ourselves—so that we can reclaim birthing and make it a unique, individual event that meets our greatest expectations and desires.

As you look more closely at your decisions, while taking an inventory of your life, you need to review your environment. It's not only the color of your child's room that's important: you will be creating both a physical and an emotional environment for which you must accept full responsibility. In many respects, the "green" way of looking at birth is equivalent to the "green" vision through which we are learning to take responsibility for cleaning up the environment; by letting consciousness, education, and empowerment inform our actions, we allow mothers and families to make great choices and to take important positive steps for themselves, the future generations, and the world today.

My goal is nothing short of creating a movement, and the movement has already begun. At one point in time, this conversation may have looked airy-fairy. You might have been considered an extremist or far too liberal for wanting to seek a more intuitive birthing process.

But given what's happening in the world and how we're becoming more aware of natural processes, learning to take better care of ourselves and our earth, and healing ourselves by integrating Western and Eastern philosophies, it is only natural for you to explore your deepest desires to consciously create the kind of childbirth you want. Just as it's now mainstream to be considerate about recycling and to choose a fuel-efficient car, that kind of thoughtfulness and the impact of where it leaves us down the road are the same as making conscious choices about your pregnancy and childbirth. It's all the same process, just another part of the same conversation. So if you desire a more conscious childbirth, no one will think you are an extremist. In fact, most of my clients are amazing everyday women and men just like you.

This book, then, is your access to this new movement, this mainstream conversation. Remember, only fifteen years ago, breast-feeding was regarded as radical; now it is the norm recommended by most doctors. Today, there are more choices for birthing than ever before, and they are becoming consistent with this new conversation. Midwives are returning to the birthing room. Birthing centers are growing in popularity. Creating the vehicles for your personal choices is all part of this movement. This is just the beginning of a global rethinking, recalibrating, and reeducating about the classic parenting paradigm.

It is my pleasure and privilege to be having this conversation with you. Thank you so much in advance for listening and offering your trust. May this newfound knowledge support you in creating everything you want for yourself, your children, your family and friends, and the world.

PART ONE

Inventing the Experience

As a woman in this culture, I have been discouraged from turning inward for answers. But sitting by the river's edge, listening to her speak to me, within me, I have come to trust my own deep womanly essence— the core of my being as woman on this earth.

My own truth lives in me like a great energy source and cannot be found anywhere else. It moves within me, prompting me toward my highest good, emerging and unfolding in absolute integrity and with complete honesty. This truth runs deep and it runs full and it runs wet and it runs free. It is as unstoppable as the river and as life-giving. It is nourishment and guidance and power. It is wisdom connected to the wisdom of all women who ever were and to the Divine itself. It is the only wisdom deserving of such a radical surrender as trust. And yet, ironically, trusting myself increases my trust in others. I know now that I can access this deep truth by taking my time and listening. And so I am, in all situations, in every time and in every place, with every person and in every relationship, a woman trusting myself.

—*Janet F. Quinn, author of*
I Am a Woman Finding My Voice

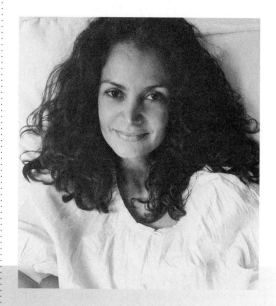

1 The BornClear Philosophy

The core goal of the BornClear program is to prepare you for childbirth on every level: emotional, intellectual, spiritual, and physical. These four key values are central to the BornClear philosophy, and they work together to help you deeply understand and trust yourself and your body. This sort of preparation can only occur when you feel completely educated and empowered to make the best choices for yourself about your baby's birth. The process begins when you recognize the deep physical and mental connection that exists within you. This is called the mind-body connection.

The Power of the Mind-Body Connection

The mind (your thoughts and feelings) and the body (your physical self) are completely connected and interdependent. Your emotions, thoughts, and beliefs affect the way your body feels on a daily basis, including the way it responds to pain. The converse is true as well: the health of your body, your respect for your body, and your ability to be comfortable with your body all affect your mood, thoughts, and beliefs. In this way, any one aspect of your mental or physical life can control or enhance another.

Dealing with stress is an excellent example of how the mind-body connection works. If you are in a demanding job or relationship, if you feel anxious and frazzled all the time, or if you always spur yourself on to accomplish more, even when you are tired, the resulting stress will eventually cause disease, or, as I like to think of it, "dis-ease," in your body. It is well documented that stress can lead to a host of physical ailments, including heart attack, high blood pressure, weight gain, and obesity. On the other hand, living with chronic or persistent pain or dwelling on and being stressed about your weight can cause clinical depression.

There is no question in my mind about the scientific and practical evidence surrounding the mind-body connection. Candace Pert, PhD, the author of *Molecules of Emotion: The Science behind Mind-Body Medicine* and many other books, believes as I do that physiology and psychology are inseparable. I deeply respect Dr. Pert's groundbreaking work, which laid the foundation for the discovery of endorphins, the hormones released by the brain (in the hypothalamus) and the body (through the pituitary glands) that act as a natural opiate or pain killer and produce a sense of well-being. From these discoveries, Dr. Pert was able to show that emotions, in the form of biochemicals such as endorphins, act as internal messengers, carrying information to link all major systems of the body into one unit.

This network of communication means that your thoughts, ideas, beliefs, and even fears about birth will affect how you experience childbirth. When you are deeply relaxed, you increase your production of endorphins, allowing for other chemicals to be released that directly influence how quickly labor comes and how comfortable you are during labor.

If you are stressed, however, or you feel fear or become upset, you increase your production of another set of hormones, called catecholamines, which will cancel out and diminish your production of endorphins. Later, I will teach you exercises that increase your endorphins during delivery, and if you do get stressed, how to counteract the catecholamines and produce even more endorphins. You will be able to use these exercises throughout your pregnancy and even afterward, for the rest of your life. If you are not pregnant yet, they can also help create the mental and physical space that will be most conducive to conception. These exercises will strengthen the internal conversation between your mind and your body so that they can work together as a unified team, just as nature designed.

The Emotions of Your Past

The renowned theorist and author Dr. Joe Dispenza, who was featured in the movie *What the Bleep Do We Know?*, believes that feelings and emotions are the product of sensory experiences. His research shows that when you are having an experience, whether you are enjoying a sunset, having a great dinner, or watching your child hit a home run, all of your five senses send a rush of information back to the brain through the five different sensory pathways. That sensory information causes neurons to string into place, which may release chemicals in your body, and those chemicals are directly related to your emotions and feelings.

Dr. Dispenza believes that if you live with the same feelings every single day, it means you are thinking in the past. Because of this, you're not having any new experiences and you're using those old feelings to determine who you think you are today. The redundancy of those same feelings and thoughts activates certain pains, which then allow specific diseases to manifest and break the body down. Eckhart Tolle, the best-selling author of *A New Earth*, refers to these "pains" as "painbodies."

By taking advantage of the knowledge and the lessons in this book, you will use your mind in a whole new way that is consistent with what you are creating: a new experience. These new thought patterns will replace your "painbodies," the "old" ways of thinking that may have left you feeling like a victim of your fears, thoughts, and confusion. You will be able to rid yourself of the cultural conversations of fear that surround you, and give yourself an opportunity to heal.

What Defines Your Reality?

In her book *Molecules of Emotion*, Dr. Pert also looks at the concept of objective reality and concludes that everyone has the ability to shape his or her own reality. With the constant barrage of stimuli from the outside world, your brain would be overloaded if you analyzed everything that you saw, heard, felt, tasted, or sensed. Instead, you instinctually pick and choose from the entire range of visual, auditory, and sensory stimuli, using a filtering system that complements your perspective on life. According to Dr. Pert, your filtering system for incoming stimuli is highly colored by your emotions at a biochemical level. Your emotions screen your experience of reality. In other words, you see what you choose to see and physically experience what you choose to experience. I like to refer to this perspective as your "context."

Your emotions also help you decide what is worth paying attention to. Because your emotional biochemicals filter so much of what you perceive, feelings and thoughts can have a profound impact on your experience of "reality." This concept is integral in understanding exactly how the mind-body connection works during pregnancy and labor. If you choose to focus on the expected pain of delivery, you will create a reality that meets your expectation of pain and consequently feel pain. If, however, you concentrate on experiencing the joy and beauty of the birth, then those emotions will create a different reality, even if the physical circumstances are exactly the same.

It's important to remember that good health and a successful, comfortable childbirth do not result merely from thinking happy thoughts. What you are trying to achieve is the optimal balance, which is based on an honest assessment of your current mental state. All of your emotions affect your body, whether you are angry, sad, or frightened. It is how you choose to deal with your emotions that will affect your physical state during pregnancy and beyond.

Through the exercises in this book you will learn to recognize what is going on inside your mind and how your thoughts, feelings, and beliefs affect not only your context, but how your body feels and how it behaves. Outwardly, you will see how you present yourself to others; inwardly, you will be able to control aches and pains or other symptoms that are currently unpleasant. Best of all, the mind-body connection might bring about positive and lasting changes. Many of my clients who have experienced BornClear childbirth feel powerful, almost invincible, for weeks afterward.

Experiencing the Mind-Body Connection

The following is one of my favorite visualizations, inspired by the book *Psychic Development* by Jean Porter. Its goal is to elicit a mind-body response. If possible, have someone read this to you so that you can be completely surprised when you experience it. Or, read through the following exercise aloud, recording your voice so that you can play it back. Before you begin, sit or lie down in a comfortable position and take five deep breaths. Let everything go, including all of your thoughts, sensations, and stresses of the day. Allow your breath to drift down through your chest, into your stomach, and down through your body into your toes. Releasing and relaxing, feel your shoulders, your chest, and your elbows become limp and relaxed.

When you are ready, close your eyes and listen to the following:

In your mind's eye, take yourself to a kitchen. This is a kitchen that you are very fond of—a place that holds good feelings for you. Look around the room. See all the familiar things in this kitchen. Feel the warmth of the room. Breathe in the wonderful aroma of your favorite food as it cooks. Hear the bubbling sound of food cooking on the top of the stove. Feel the warmth coming from the oven and the smells of baking, healthy meals.

Imagine now that you are standing at the counter in this wonderful kitchen. In front of you are a knife, a cutting board, and a large bowl full of fruit. Go over to the bowl and select one perfect, beautiful, bright, and yellow lemon. Pick it up and hold it in your hands. Feel the weight of it. Experience the texture and smell of the rind. Now, with your thumb, break into the skin and begin to peel the lemon. Be aware of the citrus fragrance. When the skin is entirely removed, feel the difference in the texture from the outside to the inside. When you are ready, pick up a small knife and cut the lemon on the cutting board. See yourself cutting the lemon in half. Watch as the juice runs down and begins to make small puddles on the board.

Now, take one half of the lemon and bring it to your nose. Smell the lemon. Bring it to your mouth and sink your teeth into the pulp. Be aware of the juices as you suck the lemon, and feel them run through your mouth. Slowly move your tongue around the inside of your mouth. Feel what is happening to your jaws, lips, and tongue.

Slowly come back to the room, opening your eyes. Take four deep breaths and think about what just happened. Did you notice the puckering of your lips and mouth; the sour taste of the lemon; the jolt of the sourness? Any or all of these sensations point out that the thought and the visual are connected by a bodily response as if you were eating a real lemon.

The goal of this exercise is to demonstrate that when you let your mind become attached to the concept of the lemon, you can cause a physical reaction. The mind actually elicits a bodily reaction. You can feel and taste the lemon. Just thinking about it, seeing the lemon in your mind, or remembering lemons you've had in the past can actually cause a real physical response in the moment, even though you are not actually eating a lemon at all. In this exercise, you can also determine which of your senses works best for you. Was it hearing the words? Or seeing the images in your mind? Going forward, you will be able to use what works best for you as you select specific exercises that enhance your understanding of the mind-body connection.

Giving Birth Consciously

One of the most important lessons in learning to control the mind-body connection is being able to create an emotionally safe space wherever you are, but particularly when you are giving birth. To me, feeling safe means the ability to relax completely, trust yourself and your personal choices, and be nurtured by this environment so that you can be fully uninhibited.

This feeling of safety is part of a universal context that every woman needs when she conceives or gives birth. Women need to feel uninhibited so that they can follow their instincts. Just as it is impossible to have passionate, meaningful sex when you feel insecure, it will be impossible for you to completely open up and release to the process of childbirth if you don't feel safe.

For many women, this feeling of safety occurs when they believe that they are in control of a situation, instead of having a situation forced on them. In the context of childbirth, safety can be achieved by choosing where you will give birth and who will attend the birth. It is well-known that animals in the wild give birth only when they feel completely safe. They have an internal system for protecting themselves that is no different from ours. Usually, animals will find a dark place that is quiet and peaceful. They don't seem to be feeling pain. But if they sense the slightest danger—such as another animal approaching—they stop the birthing process, their adrenaline kicks in, and they operate in survival mode. They then run and find a safer place, lie down, and start birthing all over again.

You will begin to feel safe and secure when you have knowledge about the birthing process and have mastered the mind-body connection. You will also need to fully understand your current fears and beliefs about childbirth so that you can begin to control both your mind and your body.

The Power of Reflection

Reflection is the second facet of the BornClear philosophy. Because the physical aspects of pregnancy and childbirth are intimately connected to your mental state, you will benefit from examining yourself thoroughly and performing an introspective study of your true needs and wants. You will be able to uncover what is working and not working about your life, and discover what issues may need to be healed.

I call this careful examination the power of reflection. By examining yourself this way, you can lay to rest specific fears or concerns that may be holding you back emotionally or affecting you physically. You will begin to understand what limits you have set for yourself, either consciously or unconsciously, and you can work on correcting negative thoughts that are standing in your way.

The process of reflection begins with identifying your current perspective, or context. Each person already exists within a particular context. Just as the mood you feel in the morning is carried through the rest of the day, your general attitude is already colored by the thoughts and beliefs you have now and have had in the past.

As Dr. Dispenza said, your thoughts and feelings have imprinted the way you approach life. In fact, each of us has already created his or her own context. If you met two men using sledgehammers on a pile of rocks, and you asked each one what he was doing, you might get two entirely different answers. The first man might say that he is breaking rocks, and the second may offer that he is building a cathedral. Even though the men are doing the same exact thing, each sees his job differently based on his life's context. They each have a completely different relationship to their work.

Everything you do at every point throughout your day exists inside your context. Every action you take or decision you make sets the tone or the perspective for all subsequent actions and expectations. These actions and expectations are fueled by your thoughts and beliefs, which create a cycle that swirls around you and which define who you are. Over time, if you focus on problems in a negative way, it results in a specific kind of personal context—a belief that everything about your life is negative. The ability to create what you want for this birth and in every aspect of your life comes from consciously designing a life to match the context you choose.

You can start by analyzing what you have already created. This type of reflection provides clarity, illuminating your current context when you look deep enough within. You think about the pieces that make up the person you are, and you reflect this person back out. Reflection allows you to observe yourself, your behaviors, habits, and thoughts without judgment. In this way you can see for the first time that your life isn't "happening" to you: you are causing your own circumstances.

Where Are You Now?

The first step in uncovering your current context is to address the negative thoughts that you've accumulated. In this way, you can arrive at a new space and start to design your entire pregnancy and childbirth experience. For example, many women approach childbirth with fear. Dr. Christiane Northrup, an expert in women's health, said that women can pick up fear the way a sponge absorbs water. There is so much fear around us, and we may absorb it in many ways—through our own thoughts and from what we read, what we see, and what we hear. We may not even realize how much fear we've absorbed. If we are not clear about the direction we want to take, it's easy to imagine how the fear around us can be overwhelming, even upsetting. But just as you can squeeze water out of a sponge, you can release your fears. Once you actually start to dismantle them, everything gets lighter, and you return to your true self.

You may have specific fears about childbirth. Youmight be concerned about pain, your past experiences with childbirths, images from television or the Internet, cultural expectations, thoughts about your body, the health of the baby, a change in your lifestyle once the baby arrives, or something more personal to you.

It's completely normal to be fearful about childbirth. In fact, the fear of childbirth is almost universal in our culture. Although women inherently know that our bodies are designed to give birth, at the same time it's almost impossible to envision how it happens. This is especially true since birthing has become medicalized and has been taken out of the world of "women's wisdom." Many of the doctors I interviewed for this book have never witnessed a birth where there was no medical intervention. This is partially because a birth without complications was never presented as part of their medical education. It is also due to the fact that for many doctors, the fear of a childbirth without intervention has become the norm. Without the knowledge of how unassisted childbirth is supposed to occur, the predominant emotion that is left for most people is fear.

Yet outside of the Western world, there are hundreds of cultures where women continue to birth their children naturally, supported only by other women in their communities. Some of these communities have reclaimed childbirth practices that were being lost in the haste to adopt Western practices. In Bali and the tsunami-ravaged Aceh region of Sumatra, Indonesia, Robin Lim, a renowned midwife, has created the Yayasan Bumi Sehat (Healthy Mother Earth) Foundation. The project trains local midwives to serve their clients by reinforcing the ancient wisdom of childbirth with the safe, culturally sensitive, gentle, appropriate application of modern techniques. If we can re-create a knowledgeable community of women, as Robin Lim has, we will be able to release the collective fears and anxieties that surround birth. It will be a new era of childbirth where the parents are enlightened, and our current cultural paradigm will shift.

I find that fear is often the result of confronting the unknown. Your fears may stem from the fact that you don't have a frame of reference for this experience. For women of childbearing age, it's quite common that their mothers gave birth at a time when women were put to sleep to deliver their babies. Even your grandmother's experience may have been similar. So you are left with fear because there is no one to share her experiences with you. Even your friends might not be comfortable enough to talk frankly about their childbirths. Or, if you have delivered before, it might not have gone the way you wanted. Without examples or information, you continue to fill your sponge with fear.

Many fears about childbirth are foisted on us from the outside. "Advice" that we receive from people, even if it is given in good faith and with only the most loving intentions, can subconsciously create new fears. For example, we've all been told that labor will be a painful experience. The fear of pain is embedded in the minds of men and women, including members of the medical community. The universal conversation about childbirth goes something like this: "Hey, good luck. You know that it's going to hurt, so I hope you make it, and don't forget to order the epidural ASAP." You don't normally hear that birthing will be a beautiful, safe, fulfilling, and even exciting experience, all of which it can be!

I always tell my clients that during pregnancy, the best thing to do is to turn off the "Birth Channel" and stop having conversations with people about their childbirth experiences, unless these are positive and uplifting. I find that it's best to create distance from others who try to impose their negative thoughts and images on us. This negativity could potentially create fear and, worse, cut off the possibility that childbirth will be a rewarding experience. You don't want to build your objective reality around someone else's story. You are then giving up the right to create your own baby's birth and instead are mirroring what the other person experienced or embellished.

No matter what your specific fear or concern is, recognize that any negative thoughts and beliefs will limit you in your childbirth and in your life. By addressing these fears and negative thoughts, you will be able to remove this attitude of fear from your current context. Just as you can absorb fear, you can also wring it out.

The following questions are meant to raise some of your conscious and unconscious fears. Answer these questions as honestly as you can, expressing all of your thoughts and concerns until you can clearly state exactly what you are afraid of. Look for common themes among your answers. For example, if you have issues with trust in general, you need to look at how lack of trust manifests in your own life, as well as the particular issues of trust surrounding your pregnancy.

- What are your current ideas about pregnancy and childbirth?
- What do you choose to think about or dwell on?
- Are you worrying about the delivery or your life after your child arrives?
- How will your relationships change?
- How will your work life change?
- Do you worry that you will repeat the same bad parenting you received from your parents?

- Are you thinking about pain?
- Are you wondering how long the delivery will take?
- Are you wondering whether you will be strong enough to recover?
- Do you wonder whether you will require medication during the delivery?
- Are you afraid that you can't deliver vaginally and will end up having a C-section?
- Are you unclear about the physical changes that will happen to your body?
- Do you understand how childbirth actually progresses?
- Are you afraid that your husband/partner/friends won't be supportive?
- Are you afraid of what your life will look like afterward?
- Do you worry about taking care of yourself and your new family?
- Do you worry that you will never sleep again?

Visualizing Fears

Another way to uncover your fears, self-limiting behaviors, or unconscious beliefs is through visualization. Visualizations allow you to see in your mind's eye what your feelings look like. This type of exercise lets you focus deeply and allows you to get to the heart of the matter.

Read through the following exercise once so that you understand it completely. Then find a space in your home where you can relax uninterrupted. Have someone who is close to you slowly read through the exercise while you are lying down with your eyes closed. Or, you can record your own voice reading the exercise and then play it back. You can return to this exercise any time you feel a need to address your fears or whenever new anxieties arise. For instance, after you have read this entire book, you will be in a different mental place than you are right now. When you repeat this exercise again, notice if the same fears or concerns surface and whether new ones crop up.

Begin by closing your mouth and breathing in deeply through your nose and out deeply through your nose. As you continue this breathing, allow yourself to relax your entire body, releasing and relaxing your jaw, gently closing your eyes, relaxing your lips, your neck—the front and the back of your neck. Imagine the same deep soothing relaxation drifting down to your shoulders, having them drop, feeling your elbows and lower arms going limp, falling heavy, washed with relaxation, your upper chest, your upper back. Use your breath to release and relax fully, caressing your body into a deep state of comfort, relaxing your stomach, letting your hips go fully, your lower back, feeling more and more relaxed as you breathe and moving that deep relaxation down and through your body. Focus on your upper legs and thighs, your knees, your lower legs, your feet, your toes. At this point you should be fully relaxed; allow yourself to go even deeper. If you hear any noises around you, interruptions, street sounds, or sounds in your home, use them to go even deeper into relaxation, giving yourself the permission and the gift to relax fully, physically and emotionally, letting all thoughts, concerns, and aches drift away and bathing yourself in this very quiet time inward, nurturing yourself, mothering yourself, in the place of your own unique essence. You are very quiet, very calm. Take a few more deep breaths and with these fall into an even deeper relaxation, releasing, relaxing, soothing.

As you are breathing and feeling relaxed, take yourself to a beach, your favorite beach, or any beach that you have enjoyed or that you have imagined. Make your beach a very sacred, safe spot where you are alone but not lonely. What time of day is it? What is around you? Take in the air, the feeling around you. Look at what you are wearing—picture yourself feeling really cozy and comfortable—bring whatever you want to your beach that will help you feel totally at ease, deeply relaxed, safe, secure. You are sitting on this beach either in a chair or on a blanket or directly on the sand. You are fully and deeply relaxed and at peace. Once you are comfortable on your beach, look out at the beautiful ocean— notice the color of the water and the waves, coming in, going out, all very soothing. In the distance on the waves you notice a clear glass bottle coming to the shore in front of you. You pick up the beautiful clear glass bottle and place it to your right on the sand.

Now look into your thoughts and see all of the images, fears, and concerns you may have about birthing your baby, becoming a parent, changing your lifestyle, stories that well-intentioned friends may have told you about their childbirths that still live in your mind. Some of your fears may be about these things, but look to see what else may be there—thoughts, beliefs, worries—and, one by one, place these images on the sand in front of you, from right to left. Lay them out. Look at them. If any other thoughts, memories, events, and feelings come up that you want to discard, face them and be free of them by placing them in an arc around your body, from right to left in the sand. Keep going through your thoughts. The mind, the subconscious, works very fast, so keep looking and placing on the sand all of the images that are not consistent with what you really want to create for your childbirth and your life after the baby's birth.

Now as you see all of these images, watch them melt into sand. Grab a handful of sand where the image was and begin to fill up your clear bottle. Watch the sand fill the bottle. Now go from image to image, morphing it into sand, grabbing it with your hand and letting it pour into the bottle. With each action, the morphing of the image into sand, your grabbing the sand and placing it into the bottle, you are dissolving that image, that fear, letting it go.

Once all of the images are in the bottle, choose a point on your ocean and toss the bottle with all of your strength. The waves are carrying away your concerns, fears, past events, and negative images. Watch as the bottle disappears and falls off the ocean's horizon, where it can no longer be seen.

Now on the sand, replace that same space with new images. See yourself now with your birthing partner. You look beautiful—you trusted yourself—you had the birth that you intended. See yourself now holding your baby, looking into your sweet baby's eyes. You did it, you created the birth you wanted, you knew you could.

Take a moment to look at this image: feel it, see it, sense it, be it. Enjoy this beautiful image fully. Add anything you want to this image to allow yourself to see and feel all that you are creating and preparing for. Breathe deeply and fully and let yourself see and feel all of this.

Count slowly from one to five, and bring yourself back to where you actually are. Take your time . . . one, you feel nourished and very relaxed . . . two, bring the feeling back into your hands and feet . . . three, begin to wiggle your fingers and toes . . . four, bring the energy fully back into your body . . . and five, bring yourself back to your room. When you are ready, and only when you are ready, open your eyes slowly and easily.

Replacing Fear with Curiosity

As Dr. Joe Dispenza said, there is a true biology to change. If you think the same thoughts and you behave the same way every single day, your brain is not changing. If you are living in fear, you will continue to live in fear. In order to create real change, you have to open up new neurological pathways by learning and experiencing new things. If you want to change your context from one that is full of fear to something else entirely, you have to combine thought and emotion: you must replace your fear with a passion for curiosity to find your new context.

A curious mind can regard these same fears or concerns in an entirely different context. You can dismantle the underlying fear by actually looking at each of your issues and replacing the fear with factual information that addresses your concerns, so that you reach a point where you are no longer afraid. Instead, you'll be educated and prepared.

You can dig underneath the fears that you bring to light during the visualization exercise by becoming curious about them. In this way, you will be able to determine whether the fears really represent your true thoughts. Ask yourself, "Do I really think that?" "Do I really fear that?" See whether you can identify where specific fears, thoughts, or beliefs came from.

Then look at each fear or concern and ask yourself how you really feel about it. Are the fears rational? I know that they may "feel" real, but by contemplating each one, you might be able to identify specific actions you can take to address them. You can answer some fears merely by reading this book and learning about the various aspects of childbirth. By replacing your fear with knowledge, you'll find that you have much less to worry about.

If you reflect on your fears, you can address them individually. For example, if you are worried about connecting with your baby, chapter 5 will help you create a bond with him or her, starting right now. If you are afraid of having a painful childbirth, the exercises in this book, particularly in the BornClear toolbox in chapter 4, will teach you how to manage pain. If you are unsure about what happens to your body during birthing, chapter 7 outlines each stage of labor so that you will be fully educated. If you are worried about how your life will change, chapter 8 will instruct you on how you can have honest and thoughtful discussions with your partner, your boss, or other important people in your life so that you can begin reflecting on the life you want to create after the baby arrives.

Working with other fears may take more effort and may require having deep conversations with yourself and with others, or even seeking support or professional help. See whether you can uncover what is buried so that you understand yourself. If you're afraid you won't be able to handle childbirth, ask yourself whether you really want to be stuck thinking about what you can't do. Once you decide that you want to be positive, you will summon the courage to take the necessary actions that will impact you positively. In this case, your first step is to get educated: reading this book and doing the exercises in it will help you deal with and eliminate the fear of childbirth. You will learn exactly how your body functions during childbirth, so that you understand what it looks like, what it will feel like, and what it will be like.

Creating Your New Context

Once you replace fear with curiosity, you can begin to create a new context. You can define what this journey *could* be like. Your reflection has given you the power to make new choices, the ones that are right for you. They can involve your pregnancy, your delivery, how you handle yourself as a mother, your life partnership, your new family, and more.

Jill was one of my clients who was able to become empowered in this way. Her first childbirth was completely traumatic, both emotionally and physically. I met her when she was five months pregnant with her second child. She was terrified that she would repeat the same bad experience again.

By working with Jill, I was able to help her rethink every aspect of her life. I encouraged her to make the necessary changes to fulfill her dream of having an easy, calm, and peaceful birth. I had her look at her last birth experience using the fear visualization. What surfaced was that Jill's brother had died in a kayaking accident about a month before she gave birth, in an area of a river called, of all things, "the birth canal." Jill did not realize that at the time of her childbirth, she was still dealing profoundly with her grief over her brother's death. So, during her second pregnancy, I worked with Jill to process her grief. She also looked at her entire life and made some empowering choices: she realized that she needed to change her job and began to research new places for her and her family to live. All of these actions helped her feel more in touch with herself.

Four months later, when the contractions started, Jill was able to let go of tension and fear and replace it with deep trust. She had a great birth and could not have been happier. The results of her second birth reflected her deep inquiry into, and courage to address, her fears. Afterward, she was empowered and educated and trusted herself. She was proud of her courage and willingness to take the necessary actions to heal and to create what she really wanted to have happen.

Your curiosity and investigation will eventually lead you to create, design, or invent the birth experience that you deeply desire. In chapter 3, you will take the next step: channeling your curiosity. For now, realize that you have taken the first important step toward creating this new context merely by facing who you really are.

The Power of Trusting Yourself

The ability to trust yourself in any aspect of your life comes from being completely educated and prepared, from taking the time to understand yourself—your gifts, your commitments, your fears, your behaviors. You must be comfortable with every aspect of the journey, which will involve careful planning, orchestrating important decisions, and sometimes having difficult conversations. Once you have had conversations with everyone who will be involved in the birth and know that your concerns have been addressed, then you will be completely prepared. I believe that this type of deep work leads to empowerment, which is the third goal for this book.

I will show you how to create distinct alignments with your partner and your entire birth team (your doctor, midwife, nurses, family members, friends, and so on) in advance. You need to not only create but to expertly write out your new context so that everyone involved knows what you want and can help you achieve it.

The first place of alignment begins at home. You alone, and you and your partner as a couple, need to create the context for the pregnancy, the birth, the new baby, and your life with the baby after he or she is born. As partners, you need to be completely aligned to get the birth you want. Everything needs to be prepared, discussed, and dealt with.

I know that it takes courage to begin this journey, to look deeply at your fears and face them. You will find that when you reflect on your fears and replace them with curiosity, when you understand the power your mind has over your body, and when you are fully educated and prepared in every aspect of your pregnancy and people around you are aware of your new context, then you will be completely satisfied with your decisions. You will have reached the fourth aspect of the program, a place where you trust your thoughts and also trust your body and then surrender. At this point, you will know that the decisions you make are the right ones for you.

For many people, this level of satisfaction is defined as happiness. All of the work you'll soon embark on is designed not only to create a beautiful birth, but to let you reach a deeper understanding of yourself. You will be better able to grasp who you are, figure out your relationships, discover what is important to you, and develop further as a human being. This journey allows you to trust yourself beyond the childbirth experience. It is an all-encompassing rite of passage because you are birthing yourself as a mother and in every aspect of your life.

Your birthing experience will be filled with many rich rewards, not the least of which is your new baby. You will also feel a deep sense of comfort once you are aligned with your partner more intensely. Most important, you will completely trust yourself, birthing yourself as a mother-father-family and more. As Erma Bombeck once said, "Instead of wishing away nine months of pregnancy, I'd have cherished every moment and realized that the wonderment growing inside me was the only chance in life to assist God in a miracle."

Let's Get Started

The BornClear program can begin as early as preconception, although whenever you begin is the right time for you. For women who have experienced difficulty in conceiving or who are merely thinking about becoming pregnant, continue the journey with chapter 2. If you are already pregnant, no matter how far along you are, you are ready to begin creating a new context with chapter 3.

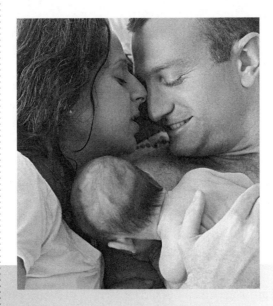

2 Consciously Conceiving

Consciously conceiving is the beginning of a holistic journey that includes physical, mental, and emotional balance. You may have discovered that conception is not always easy. Perhaps you've just started to think about conceiving, or maybe you've been trying to get pregnant for a while. Or you might have miscarried and are working on conceiving again. Each of these scenarios can lead to frustration and anxiety. Wherever you are on this journey, however, this chapter will help you begin a new process that is free from anxiety, and full of opportunities. You will learn powerful ways to create and prepare for conception.

In chapter 1, you learned to identify your current context. Revisit the "fear" exercise, replacing all of the words that refer to birth with "conceiving." You are customizing this exercise to apply to where you are right now. Then, investigate and clarify each block that is preventing you from conceiving, whether it is a physical issue or a mental or emotional attitude. In this way you will begin to design a new context, a new perspective that is empowering, so that you can use the tools in this book to help you conceive.

BornClear and Conception

Years ago, when I started teaching the BornClear courses in New York City, a couple who had registered for one of the classes miscarried the day before the class. When they gave me this news, they asked whether they could still take the course and use the philosophy and practices of BornClear to conceive again. I was a bit surprised, but I was so moved about their commitment that I said yes.

As I worked with this couple, I had them flush out and talk about their current fears and disappointments about conceiving. They opened up and shared that the woman in the marriage wasn't taking care of herself on many levels—she was intensely stressed and not eating well. She also brought up tensions that she and her husband had not resolved. Together, they began to use the BornClear toolbox on a daily basis, learning to relax and find peace. They visualized conceiving and being pregnant and then actively went to work on their relationship to resolve some of their issues and align with what they wanted to create together. They also learned about the physical process of conception and how various natural chemicals, such as adrenaline, can stress the body into an unbalanced state that could hinder conception. In addition, they checked into some of the physical aspects of their miscarriage. Out of this work and their willingness and courage to learn and grow, they became pregnant again. Then they continued with the course to create their childbirth, which ultimately went very well.

This couple made me realize that the methods and the philosophy I developed for BornClear apply to every stage of your pregnancy, from conception to delivery. Many women will come to this program once they are already pregnant. You are in the best place, however, if you start from the very beginning.

Mind-Body Conception

The mind-body connection affects conception in various ways and on many different levels. You already know that your existing context is directly influenced by the mind and the body, so it should be no surprise that this powerful link is directly related to your ability to conceive. Everything that is wrapped up inside your context, from the way you go about your day to your innermost thoughts, continually affects your ability to become pregnant, even before you "try" to have a baby. This context is an energy that grips you and creates a self-fulfilling prophecy. If you spend your days in an atmosphere of negativity or stress, your body is releasing a constant flow of stress chemicals. These chemicals—specifically, catecholamines, which include dopamine, norepinephrine, and epinephrine (adrenaline)—will directly prevent a pregnancy from occurring. Combine this physiological state with the added stress of your thoughts and fears as you rationalize why you aren't getting pregnant, and you literally exacerbate an already stagnant situation.

The chemistry behind the mind-body connection is simple. Catecholamines activate the body's fight-or-flight mechanism, in which the body gets a message to conserve resources and be ready to run away from danger. Your primitive mind is intensely programmed to optimize your survival and has not evolved in the same way that your rationally thinking brain has. For example, the primitive mind has not yet recognized that you live in a modern world and that the stresses you face every day come from your emotional insecurities and not from the fact that you might be eaten by wild animals. Yet the primitive mind still responds to stress by seeking immediate physical safety, which is prioritized over pregnancy and reproduction.

In short, when you are stressed, your body allows you to stay alive and is not too interested in letting you reproduce. Biologically, the body responds to this state of stress as your heart rate and blood pressure rise and your rate of respiration increases. The release of catecholamines also inhibits smooth muscle contractions in the gut, the lungs, and the uterus and alters blood flow to the pelvic organs. These chemicals further stress your metabolism and your hormone production, promoting the movement of body fat and blood sugar stores. For example, insulin resistance is associated with polycystic ovarian syndrome and nonovulatory cycles. Both of these conditions are considered potential causes of infertility.

Meg Richichi, an acupuncturist and creator of Mother's Path, an innovative program that embraces the challenges of infertility, has observed the escalating effects of daily stress on conception. According to Richichi, when a woman's body is in a state of constant, low-grade stress, she uses her own natural progesterone to counteract it, thereby losing her cycle and limiting her chances for conception. Richichi says, "Over the years, distinct energetic imbalances kept reappearing in my clinic. Female patients in their twenties and early thirties with non-related fertility issues were mirroring energetic disturbances of women being treated for infertility. These women were eating on the run, skipping meals, working ten-plus hours a day, drinking too much coffee and getting too little sleep. I knew from years of clinical experience that many of these women would eventually confront the challenge of infertility."

Dr. Joe Dispenza suggests that the mind-body connection further influences three distinct stages of awareness in creating new, healthy life. Stage one is preconception, stage two is prenatal (pregnancy), and stage three is postpartum. Between these stages are the literal points of contact: conception and birth. His view is that during these points of contact, you are expressing your genetic makeup in specific ways that directly affect which genes are passed to the embryo or may inhibit fertilization.

In the past, it was thought that the mother and the father simply passed on their genes to the new baby. In contrast, Dispenza believes that your thoughts and feelings at the time of conception can alter— or select—which particular genes get transferred. If the mother and the father are in a state of lust and their sexual encounter seems more like a matter of survival than of creation, then there will be a certain gene expression, one that would be very different than if they engaged in sex with the intention of creating a new life.

In native cultures such as the Aborigines and certain African and Native American tribes, the custom still exists for a couple to create a mind-body connection—in effect, solidifying their context—before conception. During this time, the partners fast and spend time alone together. The man and the woman become clear on their intention of bringing a new life into the world in a very sacred and profound way. They believe that they are inviting a new soul to enter their lives and that the act of consummation, together with that level of deep intention in the state of love, will create a good place for the soul to enter. By doing so, they are letting go of their fears and creating a loving climate in which they are completely relaxed and aware of themselves. What better way to bring a new life into this world!

Emotional Blocks to Conception

You don't have to get stuck inside a particular context that will continue to inhibit your ability to become pregnant. Instead, you can invent a new context. To create this context, you first need to uncover the underlying nature of your present situation and then address it. For example, if you learn that your stress levels are preventing conception, you will need to figure out how to get underneath your stress so that you can alter the situation. This is my definition of being empowered: having the drive, clarity, and courage to seek out the root of your issues and stay with them long enough to resolve them.

I view problems surrounding conception in a much different way than how they are conventionally seen. Far too often in our culture, the main conversations about birth and problems with conceiving are fear-based. I prefer to replace the word *problems* with a real inquiry into your own personal journey, which must occur before you conceive and which includes "life lessons." Many elements need to align before anyone can call a child into this world. Instead of dwelling on your state of fertility or infertility as a "problem," I urge you to use this time to create a unique experience for yourself. It's truly a gift to have the time to evolve and heal your life. For now, allow yourself the freedom to leave behind one doctor's opinion or the cultural conversation. It is very likely that your fertility issues point to deeper questions that you may not understand yet.

You can enter an introspective dialogue between two aspects of yourself: who you are now and who you want to be, both as a person and as a mother. This conversation needs to take place within the primitive mind. Too often, you overintellectualize issues, dwelling on what cannot be instead of creating new possibilities. You are too thinking-oriented and don't spend enough time in the body. Engaging in a dialogue in the primitive mind opens up your ability to enter the body, by locating all the places in the body where fear and stress reside.

You may have carried certain fears about pregnancy with you for your entire life, without even knowing it. For example, if you feel as if you are never good enough, you may also worry that you won't be a good parent. If you feel as if you "missed out" in your life or that life was hard, this will translate into the fertility world. Some people have a deep desire to create life, but they don't feel alive. The first step toward a successful conception, then, is to reframe your context by using the power of reflection: looking at yourself from within.

Begin by looking at the various aspects of your life. Decide how satisfied or happy you are in each area, with your friends, your work, your family, your health, your spirituality (whatever that means for you), your marriage or partnership, and your personal growth. Write down these items so that you can see the many dimensions of your life. The list will also give you an idea about which areas to work on until they have reached the place where you are satisfied with them and are at peace—and therefore free of anxiety.

Meg Richichi agrees with me that if a woman wants to mother a child, she must first become the best mother she can possibly be to herself, in every area of her life. According to Richichi, "Going inward, reacquainting ourselves with our true reflection, creates opportunity to experience the feminine face of God. We, as a species, are merely reflecting the state of our planet. We have the choice to cultivate our internal world."

One tool in the BornClear toolbox (chapter 4) is called first-thought writing. This powerful exercise lets you get to the root of your current context and provides a method to uncover what you've been thinking about. You'll also discover which emotions may be blocking you from having what you want. Follow the instructions in chapter 4, allowing ten to twenty minutes of private time. The object is to get out all of the thoughts inside your head and release them from your body.

Don't be surprised by the results of this exercise. You may see any of the previously listed fears, or others, such as "I feel vulnerable," "I'm afraid to try," "I'm scared because I'm not married," or "I can't do this by myself." By replacing fear with curiosity, you can get to the bottom of whatever is holding you back from conceiving. Remember, the things that you don't investigate are the roadblocks to your success.

Once you can identify your true thoughts and feelings about conceiving, you can change these obstacles into opportunities. To do this, you need to end the conversations that are floating around in your head and stop saying that this pregnancy won't happen. You need to resolve that you won't believe these conversations, and you will instead create a new context. You will start taking care of yourself emotionally and physically so that you not only rest your mind, but create a body that is powerfully ready to conceive.

Your Relationships May Be Holding You Back

Relationships, including the one that you have with yourself, are the barometers you use to determine your internal ease and to demonstrate to yourself whether you have a positive outlook on life. A healthy relationship is one where you feel completely free and connected. This means that you can express yourself and feel safe, loved, understood, and respected. Feeling blocked means that you are not at ease in any one of these categories when you are around a certain person or within a specific relationship.

Look at all of your relationships—with your partner, husband, parents, friends, exes, boss, and coworkers, as well as your relationship with yourself. Are they blocked in any way? Are there things you've never forgiven, upsets that were not resolved, conversations that need to happen, or resentments and disappointments that need to be laid to rest, resolved, forgiven, or all three? Are you withholding information, creating a situation where you are not truly comfortable, free, and at ease with others? Is something standing in the way between you and that person, such as unresolved judgments, opinions, or complaints?

You need to look at all parties, including yourself, in every relationship. See whether you can dissect each relationship in a nonjudgmental way and observe what is actually happening, what positive and negative aspects you are responsible for, and what the other person is contributing. Being accountable for one's actions is not always easy, but owning and admitting one's behavior can be freeing. If you understand how you are responsible for all of your actions and reactions and recognize the impact they have on others, this, in and of itself, is a deeply conscious journey and practice. The reactions that you have toward others are often red flags that point to aspects of yourself that need to heal.

Once you have looked at all of your relationships, take specific steps that will resolve any outstanding issues. Let's look at a reaction in the context of anger. First, you can sense your anger and describe why you are angry. Then, try to get to the underlying thoughts that formed the basis of your reaction. For example, you may be angry at someone because he or she hurt you in some way. Now you can look at this anger in two ways: first, uncover what the emotion triggered in you; second, figure out how to communicate your feelings to the other person in a constructive manner. I know that if I tell someone that I feel hurt, it is much less emotionally threatening than casting blame on the person or name calling. The other person is more likely to connect to my hurt on this softer level. More times than not, when I communicate like this, I get my needs taken care of. This purer level of communication also creates a safe environment for the other person to talk about and share what he or she experienced. Chapter 8 delves into this topic further as you learn to create alignment with everyone who is involved in your childbirth.

At the same time, look at your own hurt. What issue does it bring up for you that still needs to be healed? Are you reexperiencing an old wound or an incomplete situation? From there, calmly ask yourself what you really want, and try to become clear about who you are. Call on whatever resources or support you need to work through it all.

Once you address your emotional blocks, it's time to look at physical and biological conditions that may be preventing conception. It's important to do this as a second step: once you are more emotionally balanced, you might find that there is no need to move forward into investigating the physical complications. If you don't do the emotional work, you will never know whether that was the root of your problem.

Physical Issues Surrounding Fertility

Physical complications that surround fertility run a wide gamut. There may be real medical reasons why you haven't gotten pregnant yet. For example, I went to see Dr. Eden Fromberg, an osteopathic physician who is board certified in obstetrics, gynecology, and holistic medicine, when I recently miscarried. Dr. Fromberg did a complete analysis of my physical health. During the testing, she noticed that I was low in vitamin D_3, and she gave me a supplement for this vitamin that promotes greater fertility. I found out that low vitamin D levels are very common. I also learned that this vitamin is actually used in the body as a hormone and is necessary to regulate the metabolism of estrogen. Low levels can also cause insulin-resistant metabolic stress, which interferes with ovarian hormone physiology.

We worked on improving my overall energy level, which was also affecting my insulin. Here was another example of how my mood was influencing my health. Dr. Fromberg also found polyps in my uterus, one of which was about an inch long. This is a common occurrence, but who knew? Given the fact that your uterus is only about the size of a pear, an inch-sized polyp could be big enough to obstruct a pregnancy. Since then, I have had the polyps removed. In addition, we talked about how much I was working and how I could create a new rhythm for my work and home life. I reevaluated my diet: I cleaned out all processed carbohydrates and began focusing on eating a more organic diet featuring lean proteins, whole grains, vegetables, and fruits. I started exercising regularly again, including a consistent yoga practice that I love.

Dr. Fromberg has had great success treating premature ovarian failure using anthroposophic medicine in conjunction with Chinese medicine and acupuncture. She believes that there are many physical causes of infertility, including immune and blood-clotting disorders. Autoimmune disorders and genetic blood-clotting abnormalities, such as antiphospholipid antibody syndromes, lupus, and inherited thrombophilia (a tendency to clot), can be associated with early miscarriages, even before a woman realizes she is pregnant. The theory is that these conditions promote the formation of microscopic blood clots in the developing circulation between mother and baby, impeding blood and nutrient flow to the developing embryo and leading to miscarriage or pregnancy complications. According to Dr. Fromberg, these diagnoses are very complex and poorly understood so they are often not tested for since there is significant controversy about how to approach the treatment.

As you read the following material, take care that your mind doesn't spiral out of control as you worry about all of the possible "problems." The point of this section is to help you understand that just as I located the polyps in my uterus, removing any of these obstacles will allow you to create the most ideal environment in which to conceive. The medical causes of infertility can be one aspect to look into, but don't assume that these will negate your chances of becoming pregnant. You need to take everything into consideration, however, on this holistic inquiry and journey.

Medical Causes for Female Infertility

Absent or irregular ovulation is the leading cause of female infertility; nearly 40 percent of infertile women are affected by ovulatory problems. Their causes include polycystic ovarian syndrome (PCOS), which is related to metabolic insulin resistance; hypothalamic amenorrhea, which is frequently caused by a history of extreme stress, often related to eating disorders, severe dieting, or extreme exercise; and premature ovarian failure (menopause before age forty); as well as genetic and autoimmune conditions. PCOS and hypothalamic amenorrhea are complex problems that require metabolic healing through appropriate nutrition and the restoration of deficiencies, as well as mind-body practices to heal and regulate stress. Premature ovarian failure is known to respond to a combination of acupuncture and Chinese medicine; you must also adhere to detailed nutritional guidelines and support your immune system.

Other causes of infertility can include birth defects within the uterus, uterine fibroids, blocked fallopian tubes, infections, secondary infertility, and hostile cervical mucus. Certain prescription drugs and contraceptives have also been linked to infertility.

Female fertility issues are often treated with medications, minor surgical procedures (such as opening blocked fallopian tubes), and, as a last resort, in vitro fertilization. During various treatments, you may be asked to monitor your cervical mucus, peak luteal phases, and basal body temperatures. Some doctors like Dr. Fromberg will perform estrogen metabolism assessment, although most doctors do not commonly run this test, and will do hormonal profiles and timed hormonal testing.

When taken in the luteal phase and through the first trimester of pregnancy, natural progesterone can prevent miscarriages that may occur due to luteal-phase defects, in which the corpus luteum (postovulatory follicle) may not produce enough progesterone to support the developing early pregnancy. This problem is more common in women over forty but can occur at any age. Progesterone in the form of vaginal suppositories or bioadhesive gels is preferred. Vitex (chaste berry) may also help promote a healthy luteal phase. Chaste berry is contraindicated for most women with PCOS because it further raises levels of luteinizing hormone, which are usually elevated in women with PCOS.

A Note on Miscarriage

There can be many reasons for miscarriages—a combination of physical, mental, and emotional, as well as genetic, glitches. Just remember that miscarriages are incredibly common, but many women and couples who experience them don't normally talk about them. When I miscarried, I talked with many women I respected and loved. I was surprised to find out that eight out of the ten women I spoke with had previously miscarried but had never told me before.

If you have recently miscarried, please know that all of the emotions and thoughts you may be feeling—shame, embarrassment, disappointment, devastation, or doubt—are natural. When I miscarried, my partner, David, and I were so upset, first, in physically going through it, and then in dealing with the sadness and deep disappointment. But I was able to connect with the amazing aspects of the experience. We could see how strong and united we were as a team, so loving—it was very beautiful. I felt the depth of David's sadness but also his love, support, and strength.

After looking deeply at all of the emotions and physical elements that were in play, we looked at ourselves as individuals and as a couple to see whether we needed to clarify and strengthen our relationship even further to be prepared for a child. We still have visions, dreams, and signs as we try to consciously conceive again.

Remember that you are entitled to any of the feelings you may be experiencing. It is important to allow yourself time to grieve and heal. Then, you can begin to create the context for the next phase of your life. And don't forget to look for lessons and blessings in each disappointment; they will be able to point you in a direction and creation of your new context.

"My Eggs Are Rusty?"

The common fear-based conversation about difficulties in conception, especially for women over thirty-five, is that "You are too old, your eggs are too old, and this is never going to happen." This conversation is very limiting and is wrong on several counts. Although many women don't understand the limitations of the reproductive system, there are others who are spreading false information and changing the context of this conversation.

First, it is true that as we get older, it becomes more difficult to become pregnant. Fertility problems can be a result of age because egg production declines as we get older. And the eggs that are available as we mature may be flawed, resulting in birth defects or miscarriage.

The same is true for men. One study concluded that male infertility increased each year, resulting in an 11 percent decrease in successful pregnancies. As men age, their sperm declines in quality, volume, and motility.

This does not mean, however, that every woman over the age of forty will not have a healthy, normal pregnancy leading to a healthy child. Or that there are no powerful methods you can use to alter or assist your body. Each of my grandmothers had her last child at age forty-eight! Back in their day, there was never a conversation about the inability to become pregnant past a certain age: it was assumed that women could continue to get pregnant and have babies as they matured. So I feel strongly that blanket statements about "ticking biological clocks" or women losing their opportunity to have babies are irresponsibly spoken. So many pregnant women have taken the BornClear course at forty-two, forty-five, forty-eight, and fifty years of age, some of whom were first-time mothers. Most recently, a new friend, Agnes Chapski, told me while our five-year-olds were playing soccer and we were off on the sidelines playing with her ten-month-old, Chase, that she had assumed she would not be able to have a second child at the age of forty-six. So she had been really surprised to find out that she was pregnant with Chase. She attributes her conception to the ease and freedom she was feeling about her life at the time, even in the context of a very demanding career as the publisher of *Allure* magazine. This negativity toward older women also shows up when we hear that older moms are "high risk." I ask, "What is the measurement of this risk?" I had my first child at thirty-seven and my second at thirty-nine—both were very healthy, comfortable pregnancies that led to successful births.

Although there is medical data to support many of these claims, please remember that science does not hold the exclusive domain over your fertility. The issue of age has become part of the accepted norm in the medical world. Unfortunately, this fear has led women as young as their thirties to be afraid that they won't be able to conceive. Yet we all know that every woman is different. There are many ways that you can become educated to create the best results for your particular body. You are not stuck; you have plenty of options.

For example, Barbara Powers is an amazing woman who started Amayal, a birthing center in Monterrey, Mexico. She was diagnosed with leukemia fourteen years ago and chose to go a nontraditional route in her healing process. She researched her options and found doctors who were able to teach her how to regenerate all of her cells through deep emotional work. The goal was to release the anger that she knew was a part of bringing this disease to the forefront in her life. One thing she released was her own birth experience. Today, she still remains cancer free. She owes her success to creating her own new context and to her commitment not to allow all of the statistics and her diagnosis to stop her from taking her own journey. Now she has been able to harness that experience to help pregnant women create their own contexts and make their ideal childbirths realities.

Male Fertility Issues

Your husband or partner might have physical issues that prevent you from becoming pregnant. Male infertility is the inability of a man to successfully fertilize a woman's egg. Almost half of all fertility problems are due to male factor infertility, which can usually be traced to problems with producing sperm. An andrologist is the type of medical doctor your partner would need to see if you felt that he was suffering from male infertility. Andrology is a subspecialty of urology.

Men who do not produce sperm suffer from azoospermia, and those with a low sperm count suffer from oligospermia. In addition, blocked reproductive tracts, malformed sperm, or inactive sperm can be causes of male infertility. There are hormonal causes of infertility, as well as problems within the testicles themselves. Problems can exist within the blood supply to the testicles (varicocele) or in the delivery system (vas) and in sexual function. Finally, a semen allergy is a rare cause of male infertility—about 5 percent of the population experiences an allergic reaction to semen, known as human seminal plasma hypersensitivity. This immune system reaction, which can occur in both men and women, produces antibodies that kill or disable sperm cells.

Several different solutions for male infertility are available to either improve male fertility or circumvent the fertility problem. Dietary and lifestyle changes, such as taking more vitamins, minerals, and enzymes and quitting any form of substance abuse, can generally improve male factor infertility that is related to low sperm count or sperm abnormalities. There are also assisted reproductive technologies available, specifically artificial insemination and in vitro fertilization.

Artificial insemination involves the placement of sperm either directly into the cervix or into the uterus. The majority of assisted reproductive techniques (ART) now use in vitro fertilization with the woman's own eggs, which are fertilized in a laboratory. In addition to ART, there are numerous fertility drugs, fertility tests, and infertility solutions specifically for men.

Unexplained Infertility

Between 10 and 20 percent of couples who have difficulty conceiving will be diagnosed as having unexplained infertility. This means that after running various tests, a physician will not find a medical cause for infertility in either partner. It is important to remember that infertility in the medical world has been defined as not being able to get pregnant after consistently trying for one year. Yet because in our culture conversations about infertility are surrounded by so much fear, many couples jump to conclusions and worry far too early.

My first piece of advice is not to let traditional medicine give up on you and run your life, because then your circumstances will force you to give up on yourself. This is the time when you need to strengthen your faith and look for the synchronicity in your life. In spiritual law, anything is possible. There are no boundaries, and there is pure abundance. The undercurrent is that everything is truly possible once you are clear about who you are and whether you are willing to take the journey.

The Work of Preconception

Dr. Eden Fromberg suggests that before you rush to meet with a fertility specialist, you can make other important and appropriate modifications to your daily life that will affect your physical health.

These include following a nutritious diet, getting regular physical activity, and maintaining a positive mental outlook, as well as charting cycles or fertility awareness and getting adequate rest so that your body can restore its strength.

Begin by designing a new game plan: your strategy for what you will incorporate into your life in order to get pregnant. Women are so eager to become mothers, but they don't take time to mother themselves. If you create a plan and follow through, you will experience what it feels like to love yourself, listen to yourself, and be kind and compassionate to yourself. The following sections cover all of the different areas that you need to look at, in order to make changes in your lifestyle.

Cleansing and Conception

Both male and female infertility can be linked to toxins in the body and may require various degrees of detoxification. This can include abstaining from taking artificial hormones that are used for contraception and avoiding pesticides and environmental chemicals that imitate estrogen in the body.

I always suggest to my clients that before conception, each partner should undertake purification of the mind and the body. This is something I recommend for the couple, not only for the woman who will be conceiving, the reason being that the quality of sperm is also very important. It has been documented that sperm counts are lower because of environmental issues, and pesticide residues, insecticides, and other chemicals are now commonly thought to reduce male potency. Because the relationship is a partnership, the woman who will be conceiving should have her partner's support, if that is an option.

You must clear your body of substances such as alcohol, recreational drugs (while also limiting yourself to only the most necessary prescription and over-the-counter medications), and cigarettes. These harmful substances have no business being in your body when you are trying to conceive a new life. Each one can create a toxic buildup that affects all of your organs. You will want to do a hormonal detox *before* conception because you don't want toxins floating through your bloodstream after conception.

Next, choose which of the following cleanses will work best for you. Do the research to find out what each one entails and how long you will need to follow the regimen for best results. There are also supplements that can help with a chemical or hormonal detox, including calcium D-glucarate, green tea, and flax. It's not a competition, so don't feel that you need to challenge yourself to do something that you know won't work for your lifestyle. Whatever you choose, your body will thank you.

Some of the cleanses my clients have tried are:

1. Master cleanse: lemon juice, maple syrup, cayenne pepper.

2. Complete juice cleanse: green juices, wheat grass, lemon water.

3. Smoothie cleanse: packing all of your nourishment into smoothies.

4. Soup and salad diet: liquid foods, hearty salads.

5. Macrobiotic cleanse: beans, brown rice, steamed greens, squash, seaweed, avocado.

6. Raw food diet: soaked, sprouted whole foods, with their life force intact; this includes dehydrated foods that are not heated above 115 degrees.

Making Changes in Your Diet

Our hectic lives often don't allow us to sit down for, or even prepare, proper nutritious meals. I can attest that if you don't cultivate this good habit now, you will never be able to do it once your baby arrives. What's more, your bad eating habits may be contributing to your difficulties in conceiving. For example, skipping breakfast or eating a late lunch causes metabolic stress, which leads to the release of catecholamines.

Any well-balanced diet will have the proper combination of protein, whole-grain complex carbohydrates, and healthy fats at each meal, including breakfast. The best diet for conception includes foods that directly affect fetal development. To fortify the womb, choose a mixture of organic plant and animal foods, with less of an emphasis on red meats and dairy products. Choose seasonal foods that are high in antioxidants and vitamins, such as goji berries, cacao, garlic, walnuts, maca root, acai, pomegranates, and Spirulina. The goal is to increase the nutrient density of what you eat, so that every meal is packed with healthful ingredients. Stay away from stimulants like coffee and sugar, and avoid processed foods and those with additives.

Prenatal vitamins and folic acid supplementation can be beneficial during preconception. Talk with a doctor or a midwife who can prescribe the best formula for you. I prefer vitamins that are more natural. For example, I like the New Chapter Organics Perfect Prenatal vitamin, which I suggest to my clients before and during pregnancy.

Ending Chronic Stress

Chronic stress, whether emotional or physical, taxes the body beyond the release of catecholamines. We have known for a long time that stress is linked to heart disease, but recent research confirms that it directly affects fertility. Chronic stress is known to alter brain signals, as well as reduce the levels of two hormones that are crucial for ovulation. In 2006, in the *Journal of Clinical Endocrinology & Metabolism*, Dr. Sarah L. Berga reported that women who did not ovulate had excessive levels of cortisol, a stress hormone, in the brain fluid. This links directly to the mind-body connection.

Being stressed, worried, and overworked, along with not taking care of yourself and not mothering yourself, are all blocks that will not allow your body to be in the best shape mentally, emotionally, and spiritually for conception. If you feel a high amount of stress or anxiety, then you need to evaluate what thoughts you have and how they are affecting your body. Second, chronic stress can be alleviated through specific mind-body practices, such as yoga and meditation. These practices give the body and the spirit what they need: the ability to feel relaxed, nourished, and cared for, allowing for a sense of abundance and safety. These practices also decrease reactivity in the mind and the body, helping you to be more consciously aware and respond appropriately to stressful situations.

All of these practices and many more are outlined in the BornClear toolbox. Some will help you identify your current body chemistry and show you how to shift it to a more relaxed state. Others will aid in decreasing the release of catecholamines in your body. Customize the exercises and the visualizations in chapter 4 to support your holistic work. Visualize being pregnant; visualize conceiving. This tool gives you the capacity to actually see and feel what you are trying to manifest, with the knowledge that you can create it.

My clients and friends, Eli and Marla, were having a hard time getting pregnant so they began to visualize their child. They established a powerful ritual that was based in their context to begin connecting with their child. They designed their visualization themselves, and even put aside specific times of the week to do this work. During these times, they would focus on who they thought their child would be and what their life together would look like: they saw "her" coming out of a cab, laughing, and would imagine what they thought she would look like and be like, down to her features, her curly hair, her height, truly manifesting her and making space for this person to come into their lives. Sure enough, Marla soon found that she was pregnant with a baby girl, Ava. Now Ava is eleven years old and very much the beautiful girl they were "seeing" and creating. Marla and Eli credit their conception to their visualization ritual.

If you adopt these practices weekly, you can recruit your mind to defuse any uncomfortable emotions in a pinch, rather than getting upset and absorbing the stress physiologically or releasing it in unproductive and destructive ways (such as yelling at a partner or running negative mental dialogues). Doing these practices will literally change your emotions, your outlook, your physiology, and yourself.

Besides working with the toolbox to reduce your stress levels, you might want to reexamine specific areas of your life to pinpoint the source of your anxiety. See whether there are areas in your life where you may be trying to overachieve, or taking on more tasks than you are capable of completing. Overachievers are people who have already achieved but still feel the need to do more, thereby creating an imbalance in their lives. People who exhibit this behavior may be trying to compensate for feelings of insecurity and doubts about their worth.

They may be chasing unresolved issues from their past into the present, or they might be judging themselves based on one aspect of their lives, instead of the whole. If this is a word that you've heard used with respect to your career, choices, or lifestyle, it is worth examining in order to de-stress and achieve more balance. If you are putting pleasure off into the distant future instead of enjoying your life today, it may be a sign that you are being driven to achieve more than is truly necessary. *The Dolphin: Story of a Dreamer*, a special book by Sergio Bambaren, addresses this very issue. Pushing ourselves beyond the point of exhaustion, or to the exclusion of important people in our lives, can create stress that might be hampering your ability to conceive.

Take some time and examine those closest to you to see how they are living their lives. Then, reflect on how you can incorporate those same strategies in your own world. When we can put the energy that we've been devoting toward "achievement" into the truly satisfying aspects of our lives, we can release ourselves of needless expectations, and experience true, joyful peace.

Another tool you can use to alleviate stress is acupuncture, which needs to be administered by a professional. Angela Le is an acupuncturist who has had great success with infertility. When Le works with clients, she focuses on having intimate conversations that allow them to align their bodies and minds inside a safe, powerful environment. This lets people get in touch with their true essence and strength. One of Le's patients, Danielle, was on a journey to become pregnant. Not only did Le use acupuncture to help Danielle conceive, but their conversations allowed Danielle to look at her life and identify further actions she needed to take to resolve other health issues.

Meet Danielle

Danielle came to see me after trying for an entire year to get pregnant. In June 2005, she and her husband decided they were ready to have a baby. She went off the pill and thought it would be easy to conceive. By October, she began to try in earnest. But by July of the following year, she still wasn't pregnant. She had a complete battery of tests and received the "unexplained infertility" diagnosis. Meanwhile, her primary physician recommended that she see an acupuncturist to deal with her stomach problems: Danielle was having food issues that caused pain. She went to see Angela Le, who said that they could work together on Danielle's infertility, as well as on her digestive problems.

Through her work with Le, Danielle unearthed her feelings and found that she believed she was a burden to others, while at the same time she was unable to ask for the things she wanted in life. When this happened, she usually got mad, which made her push people away. She worked on learning to recognize what she needed instead and then figured out strategies for how to get it.

Danielle not only looked at herself, she also analyzed her relationships. She and her husband, Butch, began a powerful form of couple's therapy, in which Danielle was able to deal with her personal issues. Danielle felt that she and her husband didn't understand each other, so they worked on better ways to communicate. Through that, Danielle realized that one of the unresolved issues of her life was a strained relationship with her mother. This emotional state was upsetting her body so that she couldn't conceive, and it showed up in many areas of her life, such as not asking for what she needed at work and not feeling fulfilled in her marriage. Danielle then actively tried to resolve and heal her relationship with her mother.

By September 2006, things started to change. Danielle began to make decisions for herself. To her surprise, she found that her stomach problems were finally improving. In December, Danielle started to believe that she was ready to conceive. She made a manifestation board with pictures of babies and couples (see the exercise in the toolbox on page 120). She used feng shui in the house. These were small changes that began to create more alignment, internally and externally.

In February, Le suggested that Danielle go on a special diet that was yeast- and sugar-free. She began to eat healthier foods, focusing on vegetables, fish, and meat. She quit her job because she felt that she wasn't in the right place, creatively. The next week she got pregnant.

Danielle's work on herself paid off because she was able to look at every single area of her life. She stayed true to the journey and didn't get discouraged. She was willing to locate the people or the resources to make what she wanted possible. She finally felt that she was becoming the person she wanted to be. Once she was able to do what was right for her, she got pregnant within a month. In the end, she realized that she was giving birth to two people: herself and the baby.

Yoga: An Exercise for Conception

Yoga has been proved to reduce the production of catecholamines, the stress hormones that can hamper conception. There are many different types of yoga, ranging from gentle restorative techniques to vigorous exercise. Each has been noted to have its place in the work of conception.

Dr. Eden Fromberg is also the cofounder and the director of yoga programs at Lila Yoga, Dharma & Wellness in New York. She has developed Fertile Yoga, a new program that integrates vigorous yoga practice with a more gentle approach to relieve stress. Traditionally, yoga instructors have prescribed a gentle flow practice for conception. By contrast, Dr. Fromberg believes that a restorative yoga practice alone is not appropriate for all women, particularly for women who are already physically active or whose mental processes and stress levels interfere with their relaxation process. She has found that many women need a more physically challenging, vigorous practice that promotes a strong sense of accomplishment to truly release and relax. Her program integrates vigorous and cleansing poses with more relaxing and restorative ones.

Another approach is touted by Deb Flashenberg, the director of the Prenatal Yoga Center. She recommends a gentle flow practice with a focus on restorative poses that engage specific muscles and organs. For example, she would tell you to focus on exercises like the Reclined Cobbler's Pose or the Wide Angle Pose because these two postures open and soften the belly and the pelvis. She also likes to include inversions such as the Shoulder Stand, the Plow, and the Supported Plow, all of which gently compress the thyroid, an endocrine gland that helps regulate hormones in the body. This delicate balance of hormones affects not only fertility, but also menstruation.

You want to find a yoga style that best supports your journey. For example, the approach that works best for me at this point in my life is one taught by Elena Brower, the founder of Vira Yoga in New York City. Elena teaches Anusara yoga, which focuses on allowing one's heart to open and align with the body and mind. Elena's approach integrates divinity, love, and clarity, which allows me to expand on every level. I began attending these classes as part of my personally created program to prepare myself for becoming pregnant. For more information on prenatal yoga, see chapter 4.

Connecting with Your Preconceived Child

While you prepare to conceive, you can also create ways to connect with your unborn child. Many mothers, including me, have had dreams and various signs and messages before getting pregnant. Dr. David Chamberlain is one of the founders of prenatal psychology who believes in the inherent humanness of infants, which extends to their prenatal development. He has documented countless cases where parents have reported that their babies contacted them before they were even conceived.

In ancient cultures such as Tibet, China, Japan, and Korea, there is a history of a spiritual connection existing between the parents and the preconceived baby. Those countries had rituals surrounding that event, in which the parents would reach out and communicate to the baby to come and would win his attention and commitment to be born to them. When they felt that the spirit had committed to them, they proceeded to have sex to bring about conception.

What could be more meaningful than realizing that you can welcome a baby to come to you? I know that my daughter and son both came to me in their own unique ways. Before I became pregnant, I went on safari in Africa and fell in love with the continent—the big open skies and savannas. When I returned home, the name "Savannah" kept coming up all the time. For me, this name became a prominent sign. Then, when I was birthing my first child outside my house in a hot tub, I looked up into the sky, and the constellation

Orion was right overhead as my daughter was born. Initially, I did not know whether the child was a boy or a girl. When I realized I had just given birth to a girl (Savannah), I felt that Orion, her brother, who was next to be born, was showing himself and looking over us. I loved the constellation Orion and saw it everywhere, all the time, before this birth. The name initially came to me when my friend Lauren suggested it.

If you choose to listen on that dimension, there are rituals you can create to connect with your preconceived child, letting the child know you are ready for him or her. For both of my children, I led a group meditation and blessing ritual with some very close friends. We were all devoted to the child I was ready to conceive and bring into the world. My conversations with my children began then.

You can also use the affirmation exercises and the visualizations in the BornClear toolbox to create your relationship. The goal is to envision your child, your family, and your new life together. You will find that you can imagine, feel, "see," and hear what this will look like. All of the practices will take you inward so that you learn to listen in a new way.

I remember once attending a favorite mind-body workout called Intensati, created by my friend Patricia Moreno. During the last five minutes of class I closed my eyes for relaxation and cooling down, and I wasn't thinking of anything in particular. My mind was quiet for once! Suddenly, a vision dropped into my head as if from nowhere— a vision of me with my partner and my two children in a beautiful, sunny, happy home. We were all very joyful, cooking and relaxing. Then I saw a third child, but only the back of him. He would not show his face, but I felt him and felt the sweetness and joy among all of us, and I knew that this was my third child. He has not been born yet, but he has been "talking" to us and I am talking with him and listening. There is no explanation for this kind of communication, but so many of us have experienced it—thankfully and beautifully!

Since then, I've created another small ritual for this baby. I made beautiful turquoise beaded bracelets for the whole family, including for our unborn child. Each of us wears a bracelet and looks at it throughout the day.

Have fun with these rituals and create other ones that resonate for you—they will open your heart and your mind, even ultimately your body.

Ten Tips to Remember

1. Try to keep sex fun. Having an orgasm is the best natural way to help you relax when you're trying to conceive. Studies have shown that an orgasm is twenty-two times as relaxing as the average tranquilizer.

2. Don't hop out of bed right after you make love. Lying down on your back for at least five minutes after intercourse increases the odds that a sperm will connect with your egg.

3. Make love often during your most fertile period, the five days leading up to ovulation. Make love at least every forty-eight hours, to ensure that there's plenty of sperm waiting in the fallopian tube at any given time.

4. Don't turn sex into a chore. It's better to go every other day so that you can continue to put your heart into making sex as pleasurable and romantic as possible.

5. Start to keep a menstrual calendar. Note the date when your period starts and the number of days it lasts. This will also prove invaluable in pinpointing the date of conception and consequently your due date.

6. Make your vaginal environment as sperm-friendly as possible. Avoid vaginal sprays and scented tampons (which can cause a pH imbalance in the vagina), artificial lubricants, vegetable oils, glycerin, and saliva (all of which can kill sperm), as well as douching (it alters the normal acidity of the vagina, can cause infections, and may wash away cervical mucus that transports the sperm).

7. If you're monitoring your cervical mucus, do your checks before you shower, bathe, or swim. These activities can all affect the

quantity and the quality of your cervical mucus. You can also learn to check another fertility sign by feeling your cervix. As ovulation approaches, the cervix tends to rise up in your vagina, soften, and open slightly. Although it feels firm like the tip of your nose at the start of your menstrual cycle, by the time you're ready to ovulate, it feels soft and fleshy like your lips.

8. Does your partner like to spend hours on the exercise bike at the gym? Tell him to hop on the treadmill instead. A study at the University of California School of Medicine revealed that men who cycle more than 100 km per week put their fertility at risk. The repeated banging of the groin against the bicycle seat can damage essential arteries and nerves.

9. Make sure you've been properly screened for STDs and other viruses. More than one million women are affected by pelvic inflammatory disease each year. The number one cause is an untreated sexually transmitted disease.

10. Create a relaxation practice on a weekly basis that feels right to you. Call on your favorite tools from chapter 4; keep playing with and alternating the ones that resonate for you.

Building Community

You are not alone on this journey. Thousands of women and couples are experiencing the same thoughts and feelings every day. Sometimes, it's better to share your frustrations with others instead of keeping them all inside. I always recommend to my clients that they find a community that will support their journeys—whatever these may be—either online or at local meetings. I've listed some of my favorite support groups under "Fertility Support" in the Resources section at the end of the book. One of the best-known groups is Julia Indichova's Fertile Heart. She started with support circles in her Manhattan apartment and today continues a support circle in the city and holds phone-support circles around the world. She has also developed intensive workshops and other educational courses that she teaches throughout the year in many international locations, including Woodstock, New York, and London, England.

Julia's profound work, which she has documented in her two books *Inconceivable* and *The Fertile Female*, has powerfully influenced thousands of women to look at new ways to address fertility concerns. She was motivated to create this work when she was told that she was infertile. After researching all of her options and discarding the idea that she was just another medical statistic, Julia began the work of conception. She trusted, for the first time ever, that she might know best how to discover what her body needed, and she cultivated faith in her inner wisdom. Eight months later, at age forty-three, Julia gave birth to her second child.

Many of Julia's teachings are in alignment with my BornClear strategies. She instructs her clients to focus on excellent food choices, herbal support, exercise, spiritual discovery, emotional clearing, and other tactics.

She is perhaps best known for leading her phone circles. These phone conferences connect women who are all on the same journey toward conception. The phone conference is meant to be a support circle, as well as an interactive classroom where you can learn and practice Julia's unique set of tools. Julia assigns homework between sessions, but new members are always welcomed into the phone circle community.

Choosing Other Options

You may come to the realization that getting pregnant is not part of your journey, not your path. Your path for children might instead lead to adoption. Or maybe your path is to look into donor fertility treatments. You can trust this as well. As long as you feel good about your decisions and are committed to having a family, you will have everything that you want to create. What's important is that you are not attached to the process but committed to the result of a family. Only to the results.

Meet Heather

When Heather was thirty, she and her husband, Nathan, began trying to get pregnant. She said, "That was kind of like a magic number for us. We felt that we finally had health insurance; we felt that we could handle it. We had been married about five or six years and our marriage was solid so we started trying to conceive. I really thought that I would conceive in a second. I thought, For sure, this is a done deal. When it didn't work after about a year, we got a little concerned and started checking."

Heather and Nathan began to use a fertility monitor. Soon afterward, Heather became pregnant but was unable to hold a pregnancy past the first six weeks. "At the same time I started thinking that maybe there were other pieces to this puzzle. I started to find out what I could do on my own. The fertility specialist put me on Clomid [a fertility-enhancing medication], and I continued to get pregnant and then lose the pregnancy. I was beyond just accepting what my doctor said I needed to do."

Heather started taking better care of herself. "I changed my diet. I did a cleanse and other holistic treatments. I took dairy and sugar completely out of my body: I really limited meat and all animal products. I had always carried an extra fifteen to twenty pounds, and I've always been a little overweight. The doctors never said that I should lose some weight, but I felt really bad about my self-image and I just needed to do something for myself. It also put me in control of what I was eating, and I began to feel really healthy. I immediately dropped a lot of weight, and I looked fabulous, and that helped me.

"I also started going to a reflexologist once a week. Interestingly enough, my reflexologist told me that her goal was not to get me pregnant but to get me healthy. I was really resistant to her message. I felt like the goal *was* to get me pregnant. I didn't have time to wait. I wanted to have a baby. I could get healthy anytime. It's really interesting when I look back on it, but that's where I was with it."

Heather continued to see her doctor at the same time that she was doing this work on herself. The Clomid made her feel really sick. She started to have bad migraines and took it as a sign that she shouldn't continue the medication. "I did three cycles of the Clomid, and when I didn't get pregnant again, I thought, I need to explore other options. So I found Julia from Fertile Heart."

Fertile Heart is an organization that gives emotional and physical suggestions and support to women and couples who are having difficulty conceiving. Fertile Heart was giving a workshop in Manhattan when Heather first got involved. "It completely changed the way that I saw fertility," she said. "I really learned through their process that what was most important was how I felt about myself, how I connected to myself. Julia talked about dreams, reading your dreams, and body talk, which is kind of moving your body and seeing what comes up, yoga, and Mayan uterine massage. It's an old Mayan rain forest process where you do an external massage of your abdomen.

"During the entire journey, my husband continued to surprise me. Nathan never, ever gave up hope. He was relentless, and he did everything with me. He went to the workshops with me, and he would sometimes be the only man there. He would have to sing at the end of each session. He went to acupuncture with me. He got acupuncture. He went to reflexology and tried that, too. He even did a cleanse to see whether that would help."

Five years passed, and Heather still was not pregnant. "I remember Julia asked all of us one day to consider what if you don't become a mother biologically? I remember feeling completely devastated. She went around the circle, and everyone answered, and I expressed my feeling that I would die if I couldn't have a baby. So I stayed with the process. I changed my acupuncturist and started to see an acupuncturist who specialized in reproduction. She told me that I could get pregnant at any time, that she felt that I was right there. But I didn't know whether I could do this much longer.

"During the following summer, the *New York Times* wanted to do an article about our marriage. About ten years earlier, the *Times* had covered our wedding, and they wanted to do a follow-up piece. I agreed. The first question the reporter asked us was, 'Do you have children?' I said no and that is probably the one thing in our marriage that is difficult. The reporter asked me if I was willing to discuss it. I agreed to share what we were doing and hopefully it would help someone else. I explained that even though it was difficult, it was a positive thing for us that made us so much closer, and we really enjoyed the process. But when the article came out, it didn't capture what I was trying to say. It was pretty devastating, actually. The article came out on the day that we were having this huge party on the Fourth of July. All of our friends and family were at our house, and, of course, everybody knew we were going to be in the *New York Times* so everyone had bought it. It was the most difficult thing to read in print, that you can't have a child. Later, I remember telling Nathan that 'there had to be a sign. We are not seeing the sign here. We have got to open our eyes.'

"That day somebody gave us an article about Russian adoption. It was not because of the *New York Times* article, but they thought we would be interested in it. The next day we went to the grocery store, and there was an article on the front page of another newspaper about Russian adoption. I said, 'Okay, I think this is a sign.' Nathan agreed.

"We pursued the woman in the article who was coordinating Russian adoption in our area. She invited us over to meet her six children, whom she had adopted. We went there and signed up that day. We knew that this Russian adoption would be significantly expensive. But we signed up and said, "We're going to make it happen, we don't care what it takes.'

"The woman soon sent me a picture of a little boy. She said to me, 'I think I found your son.' And I was like, 'No, no, no, that's not okay. This is not the way it's supposed to happen. We are supposed to be done with our paperwork, and you told me not to look at any pictures before the paperwork is done.' She told me that if I was going to have this work for me, I needed to be a little looser. I needed to go with the flow. That's what a Russian adoption is about. You have to go with the flow. And she said, 'I'm sending you the picture because he's your son. You can look at it or not look at it, that's your choice.'

"Well, of course, I got it and I knew right away. I saw him and I said to myself, That's him. At the same time, Nathan looked at him and burst into tears. It was unbelievable. But the woman said to me, in a way that was really difficult for me to hear, 'You're still shopping around, keep your mind open. I'm going to send you more pictures.' I never connected with the other children as much as I thought they were beautiful. I knew there was something about this first child's face. I felt like I knew him. I can't explain it other than that. He looked uncannily like Nathan, although Nathan has always been resistant. He doesn't want anyone to think that we chose him for that reason. But he looks like he's Nathan's son."

Heather and Nathan moved into high gear, finishing their paperwork quickly. They were afraid that someone else could take this child. "We had to be open to the fact that he might be adopted by someone else. But Nathan was great about it. He said to me, 'If someone adopts him before we do, they are meant to be his parents. That means he'll find a home and then we have to just hope for the best for him, no matter what.'"

By November, they received permission to go to Russia to visit the child. For Heather and Nathan, it was a real journey. "My family and Nathan's family were all from Russia. So for us it was an amazing chance to go back to a place that our families had left in a bad circumstance. We arrived at the orphanage, and the baby was sleeping and the orphanage was just crumbling—smells of urine and cabbage and disgusting smells, but it felt really loving. It felt like people there really loved him. And then they brought him in. I was unprepared to see him, and I got really nervous, and I felt like I couldn't even go up to him, I was so scared. But there was Nathan, who swooped right in and played with him a little bit. He was practically asleep when we met him. He wouldn't look up at us. He was very shy. Nathan walks him around and then pops him in my arms. He immediately falls asleep. It was one of those moments, fear and love and just complete disbelief that you're in this moment where you've met your child. We bonded with him over the next three days, and then we had to leave, and we didn't know when we were coming back.

"They told us that we should expect to come back by January, but it turned out that we didn't get a court date until April. We had to return to a Russian court, where we had interpreters, and they really grilled us about him and about our lifestyle. We stayed in Russia for another month, including three weeks in his hometown and a week in Moscow to finalize all the paperwork. Then we came home, and there we were with this two-and-a-half-year-old boy who we were told would never speak, that he had poor motor skills, and they felt like he would be very delayed. There he was working our iPod after the first day at the apartment where we were staying. He was talking within three days.

"When we came home, I told Nathan that now we could stop trying because I didn't need anything else. I didn't need another child. But he said, 'How, why, why would we stop? If we have a baby, fine, then we will.' So we didn't change anything. We didn't do anything differently. In October, Micah turned three, and I never felt happier in my entire life. I felt like I was exactly where I needed to be. I was so in love with him and Nathan and our lives together, finally able to celebrate. I even completely forgot when I got my period.

"Months later, I was so nauseous I thought I had food poisoning. I was telling my mom, 'I can't believe it. I got food poisoning from dinner last night,' and I was complaining to my sister that all of these smells in New York were making me sick. She told me that she thought I was pregnant, but I said, 'No, no, no, there is no way.' I waited another week and a half to even test it because I wasn't even going there. Seven months later, after a completely healthy pregnancy and at age thirty-six, I gave birth to my second son.

"I think one of the most interesting things was that I had really learned about myself and about the kind of doctor I wanted and how I wanted the pregnancy to go. I didn't want to give up all my power in anything. I hired a midwife to help me give birth and a doula, and I just wanted to do it my way. I knew that I could, from doing the whole fertility thing; I knew that it was completely possible."

Aligning Your Intentions

At this point you should begin to design your context for consciously conceiving, using the lessons within this chapter. This context will set the tone for your journey. All of the steps you take and the choices you make within this context will help you reach balance and harmony on every level and will allow your deepest desires to happen.

I know that your journey can be uniquely stressful. Women who have difficulty conceiving suffer as much anxiety and depression as women with heart disease or cancer. That is why I urge you to use all of the great tools in the BornClear toolbox. They will help you create a practice that will readjust your internal chemistry to create the best environment for you and your soon-to-be-conceived child. There are wonderful resources listed in a section at the end of the book that specifically address your needs, as well as your concerns, so that you can find a like-minded community to share your journey with.

Your job is to stay true to your context. Don't let yourself be polluted with fear. Instead, be curious and willing to look at and create exactly what you are committed to. Remember that there are many paths on this journey, and there is no longer one single way to create a family. Allow yourself the freedom to explore all of your options and to discover and understand all of the actions, choices, and thoughts that will work best for you. You are acting not out of fear, but out of clarity, choice, and trust in yourself.

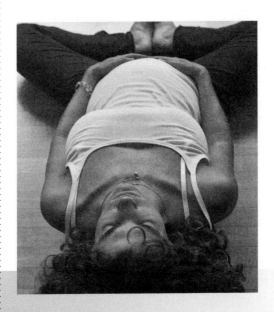

3 Pregnancy: Establishing a New Perspective

You already have a context or a perspective about everything you do in life—your relationships, your work, your body, your family—and this way of viewing things, your vantage point, manifests in what you say and do. Just as your current context creates the life you have, these same components will affect your pregnancy and birthing experience. In this chapter, you will have the opportunity to allow yourself to dream and think through what you really want the birth of your child to be like. By the end of the journey, you will step out into a whole new context for yourself, your family, and your new baby.

The universal wish for childbirth is that it be as pain-free as possible. Most women I've talked to also want to feel secure and safe and to trust that their bodies will help them have a beautiful, satisfying experience. They don't believe, however, that they can really get their wish.

They think that these are ideals that sound nice but can't possibly happen. Or, they don't know what they want or where to begin. Some new parents tell me that they wanted peaceful births and wanted to trust their bodies but then were told or decided for themselves that this wouldn't be possible, that they couldn't achieve these things. As a result, they settled on believing that they couldn't have what they wanted at all. Before they knew it, they had relinquished control by accepting this perspective, allowing themselves to adopt a disempowering collective context. I don't believe that this is how childbirth should be perceived. Instead, I will teach you how to challenge the way you think and find the courage to choose what you really want.

You are the only one who can create the childbirth experience that you dream of—and every facet of the adventure that goes with it. If you really connect with yourself, you will be able to uncover the distinct way that you want your childbirth to go and to express your desires to the people who can help make your ideal childbirth a reality.

One of the first things I teach my clients during the BornClear course is how to begin designing their context for their birth experience. This is an ongoing process: as you educate yourself, achieve clarity, and communicate with your birth team and partner, this context will become fine-tuned and unfold organically. Working through the exercises in the book will help you make your new context crystal clear. And in addition to becoming educated, you will become empowered. Then, going forward, all of the choices you make will be consistent with what you want, what you consciously design. You are completely in control: this is not about having something happen to you; you are creating exactly what you want.

Only you know what this context feels and looks like. All that you need to do is completely describe what you are thinking about. The next step is learning how to identify your deepest desires for your dream childbirth, so that they can manifest to their fullest potential during each aspect of the pregnancy. As you recognize and fully communicate what you really want, you actually begin the process of creating it.

In many ways, it's no different than building a new home. When you work with a contractor or an architect, you have to share your ideas and opinions about how you envision the kitchen, where the bedrooms will be located, or what kind of feeling the living room should have. Your ideas for your home are consistent with what your dreams are for your life within it, everything that you want to experience inside your home. The architect and the contractor can help you create exactly what you want, but only if you express your needs and desires to them clearly. The same is true for birthing. Being able to concretely express what you want helps you to get a firm picture of what you can create.

Designing Childbirth in Your Own Words

This exercise will set the tone for everything you do from this point forward in your pregnancy, including how you relate to yourself, your partner, and all of your choices. To begin the exercise, think of a few adjectives that describe how you would love your birthing experience to look and feel. They may be words like *peaceful, sacred, calm, easy, beautiful, empowering,* and *powerful*. Look for words that really describe what you would like to experience.

You may have thoughts or fears that interrupt this exercise. You may begin to see some of the things that you don't want around your birthing experience: thoughts or feelings you don't like. Words like *chaotic, hard,* or *very painful* may be associated with your current context. Write them down on another list as they come to you, so that you can address and replace them. Later, you can deal with these "unempowering" thoughts by doing the "fear" exercise again, which is described in chapter 1. It is completely normal for these fears to come up now, but just for the sake of this exercise, see whether you can put these thoughts, worries, fears, and anxieties aside.

As you think up your positive adjectives, examine the words more closely. For example, if you chose the word *beautiful*, think about what this means to you. We may all use the same words, but what I mean by *beautiful* and what you mean by *beautiful* might be completely different. Even though it's the same word, no two people have the exact same interpretation. The goal here is to find out what exactly is right for you. What do you mean by that word? What would be beautiful for you?

Maybe you came up with the word *safe*. Let's look more deeply at that word. What do you mean by *safe*? What's your definition of *safe*? *Safe* could mean that you feel relaxed or maybe uninhibited; you wouldn't care whether your clothes were off. Safe could mean comfortable, taken care of, protected, loved, or honored.

It may help to look at some magazines and pull out photos of images that convey what your adjectives feel like. A wonderful collage-making exercise in the toolbox can help you visualize and express your intentions. Another method is to think about what you don't want and then turn it on its back, shifting the negative to the positive. For example, you may not want your birth to be unbearable, so figure out what is the opposite of that. Is it *peaceful* or *fluid*, or is it sensing that you will know exactly what to do?

Continue this exercise until you have come up with at least three adjectives. Don't worry if this isn't easy for you; often people in my classes can only think of a word or two at first. But keep working on it until you have at least three words that describe what you want. Next, use these same words in the following sentences. As you do so, you are forming a complete idea about your birth:

- During the birth, I want to feel safe, which means that I will feel . . .
- I want this birth to be a beautiful experience, which means to me . . .
- What's true for me for this birth is . . .
- If I could have the birth go any way I wanted, these five words would capture what I want it to feel like:
- I want the following people to attend the birth:
- I hope that the baby experiences his or her birth as . . .
- After the birth, I want to be home for . . .
- I see a world that includes my family and my new baby, and it looks like . . .
- I choose to believe that . . .
- I want a family that looks like . . .
- My body feels like . . .

Were you able to come up with positive thoughts, or are you still hampered by your fears? If so, consider this: Do you really want to think and believe and feel all of those negative things? Or are you up for something else? As you continue on this journey, you will become more educated, and you will have more tools at your disposal to create and relax into a new context.

If you have any lingering negative worries, take each word, or feeling, and try to identify the opposite of its meaning. This process will begin pointing you toward what you want during childbirth. For example, if you come up with the word *chaotic*, try to define what the opposite of *chaotic* would be for you. Now ask yourself, do you want your childbirth to fit that definition? Continue with this exercise until all your worries have been examined and transformed into more positive words or feelings. These words should be added to your context as well.

Meet Nicole

My client Nicole couldn't verbalize what she wanted for her birth. When she was four months pregnant she came to a BornClear class and sobbed, "I don't even know what I want or what I'm thinking about!" She described her fear that the birthing experience would be "a grueling workout." She also said that she felt as if she was living "inside her head." Nicole told the class that she overthinks everything and that her thoughts made her anxious. She believed that childbirth should be a completely physical event that would give her the chance to get out of her head and into her body.

I immediately understood that Nicole's current context was centered on her pervasive anxiety. I told her that if she learned to shift away from living anxiously, she could find a way to get to peace, and she wouldn't have to worry about being anxious during childbirth.

I realized that Nicole had a tendency to rely mostly on her intellect, to the point where she shut down her intuition and her heart. I explained to Nicole and the class that because the mind and the body are intrinsically linked, we never really leave our heads during birth. I explained that having a baby is similar to planning for a marathon: When you work out a strategy for how you are going to run, you feel that you are in control, even if you have never run a race this long before. You prepare for the race by following a marathon practice schedule, which prepares you both physically and mentally. The schedule helps you develop a plan for how you will tap your internal power so that you can make the commitment to complete the race. Then, when the race begins, you enter a mental-emotional space where you trust yourself and let go, allowing your experience to be what it will, trusting that you will know what to call on when you need it.

Nicole then understood that she didn't need to leave her head during childbirth. Instead, she would be able to integrate her intellect with her body and her heart, allowing all three components of her identity to align and work fluidly together. Nicole would have to learn how to trust her body, trust her intuition, and listen to her heart, not just her mind.

Nicole could then investigate other areas in her life where she listens to her thoughts and dismisses her instincts. By learning to let herself go and trust her instincts, she would gain freedom and power—an immense gift for her and all the people with whom she comes into contact.

How Others Fit into Your New Perspective

Once you understand what you want to create, you need to convey that information. The next step is to create an alignment between yourself and your partner so that you both agree about the context for this birth. To do so, you will need to clearly communicate your deepest desires and discuss them with your partner in an open and nonthreatening way.

Sometimes men are more afraid of childbirth than women are. They don't understand everything that is happening physically. They have heard and seen grueling stories. They don't want to see their partners in pain without their being able to stop it or do anything to change it. I find that once men take my course or read this book, however, they usually realize the important role that they play. Partners can be protective, reassuring, and supportive during childbirth, which is a very important, amazing role. Also, they will ultimately be the gatekeeper of your context during the laboring process. It is really beautiful to see couples connect even more deeply through the BornClear process and during childbirth.

Two Conflicting Perspectives

If you and your partner cannot immediately align on your new context, don't worry. Be gentle with yourself and each other; most of the time, disagreements are merely a matter of getting all the information. As you read on, the answers will come. For example, Stacey and Peter were a lovely couple who came to my class. It was clear that they were very much in love, but they had completely different ideas on how they wanted their baby to be birthed. Stacey wanted a home birth, which she described as calm, quiet, sacred, and peaceful. Peter could not imagine a home birth. He could only imagine a hospital setting, and even then he couldn't come up with any adjectives that would describe what he thought it should feel or look like.

I asked both Stacey and Peter to put their individual beliefs aside for the moment. Once they understood everything about the birthing process, they could revisit their two perspectives and decide together what would be best for their new family. If you can do the same, I guarantee that you and your partner will align at some point.

By the end of the course, Stacey and Peter were aligned. The husband had learned so much about the process that all of his fears and concerns were addressed. In the end, they agreed on a home birth.

Regardless of whether you choose a home birth, a hospital, a birthing center, a midwife, a doctor, or a doula, it will be the right choice for you. There is no single right or wrong choice, as long as you are clear about what really works for you and your partner.

There are more instructions for the process of aligning in chapter 8.

Single Mothers Need Alignment, Too

Single mothers also need to create a context where they can trust themselves and be clear with their desires. They need to be able to convey their context to anyone around them, including family members, a friend, or any other support person who will assist in the delivery of the baby. Some single mothers have called on their best girlfriends to be their partners during the birth. Make sure that you choose someone who will be completely supportive and whom you can count on.

Living Inside of Your Perspective

Living inside of your perspective means that once you are clear about the context for your birth, all of the actions you take, the conversations you have, and the things you think about will be consistent with your context. Even the smallest actions need to be consistent with your overall desires. This can include how you talk with your spouse, the foods you buy, the clothing you choose to wear, or how you treat yourself during the day. You are integrating your life's perspective into your design. The more you can visualize it, the more you can feel it, the more likely you will be able to bring it into existence so that you will have the childbirth you always wanted.

What Birthing Choices Really Look Like

There are many birthing choices, and one of them will match your chosen context. Make sure that you take into account what you now know about the mind-body connection when you choose where and how you will give birth. The thoughts and emotions that come up in the environment around you can actually affect how your body will perform during labor and delivery. For example, the fluorescent lighting found in many hospitals, along with medical equipment such as blood pressure cuffs or IV stations, can make certain women feel as if something is wrong, and their labor will not progress naturally. Others might find this setting comforting because they implicitly trust the medical system and because they prefer to be close to an operating room should an emergency arise. Some women might feel most comfortable in their own homes or in a more homelike setting, such as a birthing center. Others might find these settings "too risky."

In the following pages, I outline each of the birthing options that is currently available. By reading about them, you will get a real taste of what they look and feel like. Once you fully understand each option, you will be educated about your choices so that you can identify the best match for your context. I hope I can dispel some of the myths surrounding these options and clarify certain terms that are thrown around quite irresponsibly regarding each of them. My goal is to create awareness based on facts, allowing people to be broad-minded about all of their choices.

There is more to learn in later chapters. Be aware that you can and possibly will change your mind at any point. I once worked with a woman who took the course in her ninth month of pregnancy, completely determined to have a hospital birth. She became so clear and knowledgeable, however, that she realized that her original choices for childbirth would not work for her. She discovered that she was not connected to her doctor and still had many concerns about their lack of communication and difference of philosophy. After the course, even on such short notice, she chose an entirely new birth plan and decided to give birth at a birthing center. Within two weeks, all of the details were handled. She was so much happier and calmer and as a result had a great birth experience.

Defining *Natural Childbirth*

Natural childbirth is based on the understanding that your body is designed for birthing and that bringing a child into this world is a normal, natural process. Inherently, people who believe in natural childbirth do not view birth as a medical procedure. Instead, we believe that the mother plays an active role. The BornClear definition of natural childbirth is the understanding that nature has provided many amazing tools: intuition, a knowing body, and your internal chemicals, all of which can be called on during a normal birth. As you read the rest of this book, your definition of *natural* will become clear. You can have a natural childbirth in any setting you choose: hospital, a birthing center, or at home.

A Hospital Birth with Doctors and Nurses

A hospital birth may be a necessary choice if you have a chronic medical condition that requires regular medication, such as diabetes, hypertension, a seizure disorder, or severe asthma. Over the course of your pregnancy, your physician will periodically assess the well-being of your pregnancy in an effort to rule out complications such as preterm labor, placenta previa, preeclampsia, and pregnancy-induced hypertension. In the event that complications do develop during the pregnancy, a hospital may then become the best place for your baby to be born.

When looking at this option, you are actually making two decisions. The first is whether you are connected and comfortable with your current obstetrician. The second is whether you feel connected and safe at the hospital he or she is affiliated with. You need to understand your doctor's philosophy on childbirth and feel at ease enough to ask him or her all of your questions. You will also need to be clear on the standard procedures and policies at the hospital. Chapter 8 lists the questions to ask and the issues you need to cover in order to align with your doctor and at the hospital.

It is so hard to generalize about doctors and their philosophies, except to say that in the course of writing this book, we interviewed many obstetricians who told us that in medical school and even up until the present, many of them had never see a normal, natural, unassisted birth. This means that for many doctors, their context for birth includes some level of intervention. Although it is true that a doctor's formal medical education is more extensive in the area of obstetrics, obstetricians are not necessarily more experienced than midwives when dealing with normal labor and birth. Dr. Michael

Rosenthal, a retired obstetrician in Upland, California, admitted, "I didn't learn about women in childbirth by going to medical school but rather by watching women giving birth normally." He added, "Doctors are trained to intervene."

Dr. Marsden Wagner added, "Generally speaking, a fundamental difference between midwifery care and physician care at birth has to do with control. Doctors 'deliver' babies and believe that having a baby is something that happens to a woman. Midwives assist at birth and believe that giving birth is something a woman does."

Every hospital has its own procedures, which fall within a certain range of expectations. For the most part, hospitals today have a wing devoted to the care of both the mother and the baby. This department is filled with obstetricians and gynecologists, along with pediatricians. It is also staffed with nurses who specialize in these areas, as well as physician specialists (that is, neonatal doctors, surgeons, and so on).

Many hospitals offer "birthing rooms" that unlike typical hospital rooms are cozy and homelike. Mothers will deliver their babies in these rooms. Birthing rooms are usually private, but sometimes you might have to share a room. The birthing room will have space for a birthing chair for you (and often a recliner for your partner). If you deliver vaginally, you will stay in the birthing room until the baby is delivered. Then you may be moved to another room for the remainder of your stay, usually two days.

If you need to have a Cesarean section or if there are other complications, you will be moved to an operating room. (See chapter 7 for more about C-sections.) Your spouse or partner will be allowed to accompany you during the delivery, but only after the anesthesiologist has administered the anesthesia. Once you are out of the O.R., you will recover for a short stint of time in a recovery room. This period usually lasts about two to four hours, often only until the anesthesia wears off. Afterward, you will be moved to a postpartum room for the duration of your stay, which is usually four days.

Hospital policies and automatic procedures could include the following standard practices. Once you enter the hospital, you will be hooked up to a fetal monitor that measures the baby's heartbeat in

relation to your contractions. You may also be connected to an intra-
venous drip (IV) or at the very least have a hep lock placed (a small
tube connected to a catheter in your vein to allow quick access if an
IV becomes necessary). Your doctor or a hospital intern will check
on your internal physical changes according to a schedule: they will
not stay with you from the moment you get to the hospital until the
birth. Often, the doctor is not called to attend until you are close to
delivery. A nurse will also check in with you, on a schedule. You may
be offered various medications, including an epidural and Pitocin,
to facilitate the process of labor. (This process is explained in more
detail in chapter 6.)

When your cervix has fully dilated and the baby is ready to be born,
a doctor and at least one nurse will attend and assist for the birth.
Your spouse or partner will be allowed to stay in the room for the
birth. After delivery, the baby will be given to you immediately and
then will be removed from the room to the nursery for initial identifying and a neonatal exam, unless the hospital practices true rooming
in. In this case, the baby exam, if requested, can be done in the room
with the parents as long as the baby's condition is stable. Afterward,
the baby will be returned to you once you are moved to your new
location.

Then, you can request that the baby "room in" with you. Or, you
can choose to have the baby remain in the nursery, where she will be
attended to by the nursing staff and fed, if you choose not to breast-
feed. If you plan to breast-feed, you might find it easier for the baby
to stay with you. Otherwise, the nurse will bring the baby to you
when she needs to nurse.

One of the drawbacks of a hospital birth is that when you are in a
hospital, you are following a schedule, either the caregiver's (doctor's)
clock or the hospital's time clock. This fact is not often spoken about.
There are also many rules and regulations that hospitals need to follow, some of which have nothing to do with you. They exist to meet
insurance requirements and can be very limiting to the experience you
may want to create. Some hospitals and doctors are more flexible than
others about these rules. I encourage my clients to become familiar

with some of the clinical parameters of labor management. Questions that you should ask your doctor include:

- How long will my pregnancy be allowed to continue before induction for post dates is considered?
- If my water breaks first, what happens next?
- Is there a period of time where my body will have a chance to begin labor on its own?
- At what point will my labor be induced and with what?

Meet Kathryn and Josh

Kathryn and Josh were in their late thirties when she became pregnant with their first child. They had planned to give birth in a birthing center and were excited about doing it naturally. Kathryn's water broke one Saturday night before Christmas. She called her doctor, who told her to come into his office in the morning to do a stress test; because she was thirty-seven, he had labeled her at moderately high risk. She had mild contractions throughout the night, but by the time she arrived at the doctor's office, the contractions had slowed. Later in the day, the contractions totally stopped. Kathryn and Josh knew that the protocol for the birthing center was that she would need to be in active labor for twenty-four hours after her water broke, so they realized that the birthing center was no longer an option for them. Instead, they listened to their doctor and headed for a delivery in the hospital.

Initially, Kathryn was angry and frustrated at this change in plans. She was crying when they arrived at the hospital. The doctor told her that the hospital's policy was to start Kathryn on Pitocin. Kathryn was upset, thinking that Pitocin would lead to an automatic epidural, and she did not want either. But she reexamined her thinking and adjusted her perspective. By 11:00 p.m., the nurse gave her a Pitocin drip. Around 3:00 a.m., she began to feel slight contractions, and by 5:00 a.m., she was having very intense contractions. She was soon about 4 centimeters dilated but in intense pain from the Pitocin, without experiencing any pain relief. She agreed to the epidural as well as a catheter for her urine. Kathryn began to use some of the toolbox exercises to calm herself down and accept that this birth did not look like what she had intended or even prepared for. At the same time, she realized that she still had a choice about how she would deal with the situation at hand. Around 6 p.m., she felt the urge to push. This was an interesting sensation, given that she could not feel her legs or lower abdomen. She got creative, and, with the support of Josh and a nurse, she asked to be held in a squat so that she could better act on her urges to push. When a woman is in a vertical position (sitting, squatting, or standing), more blood and oxygen get to the baby, the woman's pelvis is more open to let the baby out, and the woman is giving birth downhill instead of uphill against gravity as she would be if she were on her back. A few hours later, she pushed her baby out and received her fully with love.

Understanding a Doula's Role

Doulas are advocates for the mother or the couple during the birthing process. They offer emotional and physical comfort and informational support to families when the women are in labor. Most have received specific training and certification, although some have not. Doulas offer only nonmedical care. It is a job that does not require any medical background: fewer than 10 percent of them were in the medical field before they became doulas. Many new mothers who have used doulas come away from the childbirth feeling empowered, and they describe their birth experience as wonderful.

Doulas are valuable in any birth setting. It has been found that when a doula is present in the hospital birthing room, there are often fewer requests for medication and a decreased use of forceps. Some studies show a drop in the Cesarean rate by as much as 15 percent. Doulas do not facilitate a particular type of birth but rather help the couple have the birth they want. Doulas can also be a great reminder of the birthing context that you have created, and they will lovingly support you throughout the childbirth. They offer continuous physical, as well as emotional, support and help with pain-management techniques. They are available to explain the pros and cons of various medical or natural birthing procedures and to reassure new parents that labor is progressing normally. Sometimes they are there simply to offer a hand to hold or to massage the mother-to-be. Physically, a doula will help you get up and move, will rub your back and your feet, and will teach your partner to do all of these things for you as well. Doulas can offer suggestions on birthing positions or various pain-management techniques that you might not already know. Most important, their job is to be present, attentive, encouraging, and supportive.

A doula is hired before the birthing mother goes into labor. The doula often builds a relationship with the new mother and the couple before the delivery, allowing them to trust themselves and feel emo-tionally supported, safer, and taken care of, which in turn will affect the mother's body during delivery.

A doula can also:

- get you to the hospital and help you check in.
- update your family and friends during the delivery.
- keep your birth plan on track (see chapter 8).
- take a walk with you during labor.
- act as a labor coach.
- take pictures.

A Hospital Birth with Doctors, Nurses, and a Doula

A doula can attend a hospital birth along with your partner. If you are interested in having a doula attend your birth, you will need to find out whether the hospital you have chosen allows this. If not, then you will need to choose another hospital. Some doctors are very much against doulas, while others adamantly feel that doulas make their job easier.

In a hospital setting, a doula remains in the delivery room dur-ing the entire birth and becomes a part of every conversation. She is your representative to the hospital staff and will advocate for your wishes and your partner's. Doulas also offer emotional support in the hospital to both the mother and the partner. Your partner obviously wants to be everything he can, but if this is your first child, most likely your partner hasn't gone through this before, and he doesn't have the background that a doula has. The doula works with your partner to help him be the best support he is capable of being. The doula can remind him to massage you, hold your hand, or just be present with you.

Doulas also supply information when there are medical issues and decisions to be made. For example, if complications of any sort occur, a doula will listen to the suggestions being made by the doctor, and will inform you of the pros and cons of each choice. The doula does not choose what you should do. Because doulas have witnessed many births, however, they offer an intelligent point of view consistent with your birthing context. In that way, doulas act as advocates and gate-keepers during the delivery.

Meet Sophia and David

Sophia and David gave birth naturally to their son in a hospital with their doula, Nicole.

On Friday, Sophia went to the doctor's office, and she was 2 centimeters dilated. She had lost her mucous plug, with a slight bloody show but no noticeable contractions. On Monday night, Sophia had slight cramping with back pressure. She called her doula Tuesday morning and told her that the contractions were about ten minutes apart. At 7:00 p.m., Sophia's contractions occurred every five minutes. By this time, Nicole was at the couple's house and assisting Sophia into various labor positions, which included squatting and walking, Nicole also massaged Sophia's feet and lower back, applied counterpressure to the top of her hips during contractions, gave her water and snacks, and emotionally reassured her in a peaceful, loving way. Sophia wanted to be in the bathtub, so Nicole assisted Sophia in getting in bathtub, while David prepared to take everyone to the hospital. When Sophia arrived at the hospital, there was no bed available.

Nicole was able to keep Sophia calm until a room was prepared. When they got into the room at 10:30 p.m., Sophia was about 8 to 9 centimeters dilated. She kneeled on the floor, Nicole kneeled with her, and they rocked back and forth. Sophia's partner, David, was massaging her back. Nicole and David took turns supporting Sophia's body, and by 11:00 p.m. she was fully dilated. She pushed for about an hour and twenty minutes and gave birth to their baby boy. Nicole assisted Sophia with the initial breast-feeding. Sophia looked so elated and profoundly happy; it was apparent that this experience was perfect and priceless for her.

Understanding a Midwife's Role

Midwives recognize that pregnancy and birth are natural and normal processes—but midwives are open to using medical intervention when and if necessary. They look at birth from a holistic vantage point, taking into consideration the physical, emotional, and mental states of their clients. Midwives consider themselves the guardians of normal birth, often placing great emphasis on reducing unnecessary interventions (such as C-sections) and enhancing the psychological empowerment of the birthing family. They describe their role as "catching" the baby, not "delivering" it, because the mother is the one doing the work.

Midwives play an essential role in maternity care and are valued health-care professionals, both in highly industrialized countries and in developing countries. They are first and foremost birthing professionals, many of whom have formal medical education and training, even though they are not doctors. Although there are distinct differences between doctors' and midwives' scope of practice, the crux of the differentiation lies more in their philosophical approach to birth than in their various skill sets.

Midwives have been well trained to deal with a host of complications. Midwifery is legally recognized in one form or another in all but ten U.S. states and the District of Columbia. The states that prohibit midwifery are Alabama, Illinois, Indiana, Iowa, Kentucky, Maryland, Missouri, North Carolina, South Dakota, and Wyoming.

Midwives are often part of the clinical staff at a hospital or a birthing center, or they might own and operate a private practice with privileges to "catch" in any setting (a hospital, a birthing center, or at home). Midwives do not perform Cesarean sections or instrumental deliveries, nor do they routinely care for high-risk pregnancies. If interventions become necessary, the consultant physician will be called on to perform them.

Midwives who practice in the United States fall into three distinct categories, and your ability to choose among them varies greatly according to where you live. Certified nurse midwives are registered nurses who attended additional schooling (up to seven years in some states) through approved programs of the American College of Nurse Midwives (ACNM). They can "catch" babies in any setting: hospitals, birthing centers, or at home. Nurse midwives are formally recognized by the American College of Ob-Gyns (ACOG) and are licensed in all fifty states. At this point in time, all nurse midwives need a formal agreement with consultant physicians stating that the latter agree to be available in the event that a pregnancy or a labor becomes a high risk. In a doctor's office or a hospital setting, nurse midwives can write prescriptions and request lab work: they can do everything that a doctor can do except perform C-sections. They are like nurse practitioners but for obstetrics.

A second category is licensed, certified, or direct-entry (non-nurse) midwives, who can practice in a home or a birth center. They receive their training through a combination of formal schooling, correspondence courses, self-study, and apprenticeship. A third category is lay or empirical midwives. They are also considered to be direct-entry midwives, who obtain their training through a variety of routes. These midwives can also have practices with their clients in hospitals, in birthing centers, and at home, and they have relationships with doctors for possible medical procedures that may be necessary.

A nurse midwife or direct-entry midwife transferring a woman in labor to an obstetrician is analogous to a family physician referring a patient to a specialist, like a surgeon. It does not mean that the family physician is not competent, only that the surgeon has a different expertise—an expertise in handling specific complications. The relationship should be an active collaboration based on mutual respect between health professionals of equal standing.

Midwives monitor the physical, psychological, and social well-being of the mother throughout pregnancy, as well as during labor and delivery. They provide the mother with individualized education, counseling, prenatal care, continuous hands-on assistance during labor and delivery, and postpartum support. This woman-centered model of care has been proved to reduce the incidence of birth injuries, traumas, and Cesarean sections.

One of the fundamental differences between midwives and doctors is how they view pregnancy and birth. Midwives typically call the women in their care "clients," not "patients." Midwives work hard to build close relationships with their clients and their clients' families. During prenatal visits, they spend much more time with each woman than an obstetrician would. Women also count on their midwives to be present from the beginning of labor until after the birth.

It is just as important for you to feel connected and comfortable with a midwife as it is with a doctor. You will need to interview the midwife at your first meeting; ask questions until you are clear on all aspects of this type of birth. You may want to know how many years the midwife has been practicing, what her philosophy is, how many births she has attended, and so on. Because midwives offer a different, more intimate kind of care, make sure that you find one who makes you feel comfortable in every way. Do you have a stomach cramp when you talk to her? Or do you feel better and find yourself relaxing inwardly and feeling at ease while she talks to you? Do you feel as if you're going to have to perform during childbirth? Would you be able to have a bowel movement in front of her? Does she have a grating voice or presence? These are the kinds of things you need to find out.

Many women feel encouraged and empowered when they give birth with a midwife present. Often, new mothers find that they get in touch with their intuitive nature and the privilege, power, and divinity of being a woman.

— *Ina May Gaskin: A Midwife's Midwife* —

Ina May Gaskin is a legendary midwife, who has been practicing as a certified professional midwife (CPM) since the early 1970s, and the author of *Spiritual Midwifery* and *Ina May's Guide to Childbirth*. Her first child was born in a hospital, and she was not exactly inspired by her experience. When she was ready to have a second baby, she was fortunate to meet other women who refused to go to hospitals to give birth. The experience was so life-changing that afterward, she began to devote her life to midwifery. She said, "It was the first time there was a profession that I was interested in."

Later she settled in Tennessee, pooled her resources, and bought a big piece of land, where she still runs the now-famous Farm Midwifery Center. It trains midwives from all over the world and offers a place for women to come for a home birth outside of their own homes. Over the years, she has kept excellent records of every one of her center's births and has found that its rates of normal, natural births have been higher than in hospitals, in many respects. Ina May also developed the Gaskin Maneuver. The first obstetrical maneuver to be named after a midwife, it embodies the essence of midwifery by using simple body movements to facilitate a difficult birth.

Ina May described for me what she views as a typical midwife birth. In her words, "a midwife birth looks completely different than a hospital birth. The woman who is gently mothered by a midwife or nurse through her labor learns some of the most important skills she will need as a parent. It has become more evident that the return of the birthing process to women is important to society at large, not just to the women and children involved. The way babies are treated at birth is likely to affect them forever. The way women are treated during childbirth affects them in all their relationships for the rest of their lives.

"First, the birthing woman will not be asked to lie down on a bed when she is in labor. She is going to be up moving around, constantly changing positions. She has a lot of choices about how she spends the time right before labor, instead of being in a fixed position accommodating herself to the monitoring equipment in a hospital. At a home birth, you are not on anyone else's time clock. If a mother's vital signs are good and a baby's vital signs are good, we continue until the baby is born. At a home birth, you can eat. Also, the midwife is in a room with the mother at all times, so they can keep a close eye on her because she has human contact all the way through."

The sociologist Barbara Katz Rothman describes the midwife's philosophy in these words: "It's not just the making of babies, but the making of *mothers* that midwives see as the miracle of birth."

A Birthing Center Birth with Midwives

A birthing center is a medical facility, often associated with a hospital, that is designed to provide a comfortable, homelike setting during childbirth and is generally less restrictive than a hospital in terms of its clinical management protocols. In many birthing centers, there are no routine IVs being inserted into prospective mothers and there is less fetal monitoring, as well as more relaxed institutional regulations, such as allowing family members or friends to attend the delivery. The mother also has more freedom to move and change positions.

Birthing centers can be run by hospitals, individual obstetricians, or midwives. For women who have low-risk pregnancies and want more natural birth experiences, a birthing center might be a good choice. Doulas may be allowed to attend a birth at a birthing center; check your local birthing center to see what its particular rules are.

Usually, birthing center personnel will not induce or augment labor with drugs such as Pitocin. External fetal monitoring is done intermittently with a hand-held Doppler (a diagnostic, low-intensity ultrasound that detects blood flow in arteries or veins), instead of continuously, and no drugs are offered for pain relief except local analgesia for suture tears after delivery. Medications are available if you request them. Birthing centers are equipped to deal with certain complications and for that purpose usually have an array of medications to stop a hemorrhage, IVs that can be put in quickly in the event of a hemorrhage, and neonatal resuscitation equipment such as oxygen, suction, and Ambu bags, much like most home-birth midwives have. Birthing centers, however, often have as high as a 30 percent transfer rate (sending the mother to a hospital to deal with complications). In a birthing center, the mother can return home shortly after the birth; there is no set schedule as compared to the rules in a hospital.

Birthing center personnel perform very few episiotomies and are not allowed to perform any operative deliveries: if you require a Cesarean section for any reason, you will have to leave the birthing center and be transferred to a hospital. Because many birthing centers are within or near hospitals, this is usually not a problem. In fact, if the birthing center is connected to a hospital, medical intervention can be initiated more quickly, but it always involves transfer to a regular labor and delivery unit.

It is always best to research birthing centers in your area to find the one that suits your perspective and context. If you choose a birthing center connected to a hospital, ask whether it has its own staff or is staffed by hospital personnel. You may also want to know in which situations the birthing center would obtain the assistance of hospital personnel and how often this occurs. You will want to understand the inner workings of the birthing center you choose: its procedures, guidelines and rules, philosophy, and relationship with a hospital or doctors if you have to be transferred. Know that as warm, nurturing, and intimate as a birthing center can be, it may still have rules and regulations it needs to follow. You need to understand all of this. Sometimes at birthing centers there is a team of midwives that rotates, and, depending on when you go into labor, you may have no control over choosing the midwife who attends your birth.

Dr. Jacques Moritz operates the birthing center at New York City's St. Luke's–Roosevelt Hospital. His birthing center is run by midwives, and doctors are called in only to assist certain birthing complications, such as those that require Cesarean sections. Dr. Moritz believes that this system makes the most sense and is the most cost-effective because the midwife does what she knows best, which is assisting natural, normal birth and taking care of women. Then the doctors are able to do what they do best, which is intervening if there are complications, recognizing when they need to intervene, and knowing how to manage the complications to support the midwife.

Dr. Moritz admits that many doctors find birthing centers and midwives to be threatening. This might be because doctors are trained in treating high-risk pregnancies and often never learn what to do during a normal vaginal delivery. So their thinking is that even in the most benign situations, a disaster may be waiting to happen and their training will be necessary. As you can imagine, though, for the majority of pregnancies, this is not the case.

Meet Karen

Karen had two children who were both born in a traditional hospital setting. After each birth, she felt disappointed with the entire process. In the hospital, she was forced into a certain pattern that made her feel that a medicated birth was inevitable. It was recommended that she stop eating, so her blood pressure was low; the baby's blood pressure also dropped, which meant Karen had to be put on an IV. Consequently, she couldn't move around very much. Next they monitored the heartbeat, causing the contractions to slow down. This necessitated Karen taking Pitocin to stimulate them. With all of these combined factors—the elevated levels of stress caused by the Pitocin, not being able to move, the constant monitoring, and people coming in and out of the room—Karen couldn't relax enough for her cervix to dilate.

When she was pregnant with her third child, she decided to give birth in a birthing center within a hospital. She felt that a birthing center offered all of the options she was looking for: she would be able to have a more natural childbirth, but still have the safety net of knowing that an epidural was just one floor away. Karen interviewed midwives and was able to convince her husband that she would be safe with this level of care.

She then began to use the BornClear methodology and reported that she was "completely prepared, whereas prior classes didn't leave me feeling ready for the birth. There was something about preparing that made me feel more capable. This time, I had the feeling that I was doing workouts that would get me ready.

"On the day I delivered, I felt this underlying current of concern that I just wouldn't open. In my last two pregnancies, I could not relax enough to dilate beyond 1 or 2 centimeters. So I was very concerned that when I got to the birthing center, I would not be dilated and again would have to resort to medical intervention. So when I did get to the hospital and I was only about 2½ to 3 centimeters, I thought, Here we go again. I took the midwife's advice and just walked around outside, and by the time I got back, I was in pain from the contractions. The midwife on staff pronounced me 6 centimeters dilated, at which point I could feel nothing. It became easy. It became natural. I could be comfortably relaxed because my mind was no longer in the picture, saying, You see, you can't do it, you can't do it."

Karen felt that the birthing center environment supported her context and her intentions for the birth. She was able to tap into her own strength and quiet mind. And because there wasn't a constant flow of people in and out of the room, the peacefulness gave her a feeling of safety so that she could just relax.

A Home Birth with Midwives (with or without a Doula)

Home birth is no longer considered to be "alternative" or part of the lunatic fringe. Just look at the recent documentary *The Business of Being Born* by Ricki Lake and Abby Epstein, or at *Birth*, an audio documentary created by Tania Ketenjian and Ahri Golden of Thin Air Media, or at the play *Bold* by Karen Brody. Famous home birthers include Pamela Anderson, Cindy Crawford, Ricki Lake, Demi Moore, Kelly Preston, and Meryl Streep. Women across the country, and the world, are deciding that this less conventional route is a more personal, and possibly safer, way to birth their children. Many women who have given birth in hospitals and were not satisfied with the experience are seriously evaluating the home-birth option. Some advantages of a home birth are greater intimacy between family members; the privacy of the event for the mother, thereby decreasing her inhibitions; and the opportunity to have time to discover one's own natural responses to labor and birth.

Dr. Marsden Wagner is a tremendous supporter of midwives and home birthing. He was trained in pediatrics and obstetrics in a very orthodox way in medical school at University of California–Los Angeles. He later became the director of women's and children's health at the World Health Organization (WHO). He was stationed in Copenhagen, Denmark, in that capacity when he first discovered midwifery. His first viewing of a home birth was an absolute epiphany. He told me, "I was absolutely stunned as I watched this woman get her power and take a hold of the birth, take a hold of her body and it was clear—I witnessed for the first time in my life, a woman in her full power."

Since then, Dr. Wagner's work has been about supporting this thinking and about trying to change the paradigm of women, as well as of doctors. At WHO, he created a study group that looked at all of the world's literature and took a survey of alternative birth practices around the world. The study found that there is absolutely no scientific evidence proving that a planned home birth is more dangerous than a hospital birth. A second study by the *British Medical Journal* collected data from more than five thousand women who were planning home births in the United States and Canada and found that outcomes for mothers and babies were the same as for low-risk mothers giving birth in hospitals but with a fraction of the interventions. The study concluded that there was ample evidence to show that being in labor at home increases a woman's likelihood of having a birth that is both satisfying and safe.

A home birth looks totally different from a hospital birth and is even very different from a natural birth at a birthing center. The mother has more control over her surroundings and can eat and move around. She is often more comfortable in her own home, and increased comfort contributes to shorter labor. Here again is where the mind-body connection comes into play: if you are more comfortable and relaxed, your labor and delivery can go smoother and will have fewer complications. There are no arbitrary institutional time constraints with a home birth—you can labor calmly with no external pressures or interruptions. Most important, you can control your entire environment. Home births are attended by a midwife and often a doula as well.

For many women, the perceived risks of a natural home birth are far outweighed by the risks of hospital deliveries, where C-section rates are high, and there are many incidences of hospital staff members distributing the wrong medication or the patient getting infections. If a complication arises during a home birth, you will have to be quickly moved to a hospital. The midwives who attend home births, however, are fully prepared for most complications. They bring with them a number of the medical accoutrements that hospitals use, including an IV, an oxygen tank, Pitocin, a Doppler, clamps, sutures, and sterilized needles. In addition, before the birth the midwife always devises a plan in case the new mother needs to be transferred to a hospital. The ACNM wisely recommends that home birth take place within a thirty-minute distance from a back-up hospital, which is in keeping with hospital protocols for sufficient preparation for a C-section.

At a home birth, a doula supports the mother in the same non-medical ways that she would in a hospital. Doulas offer comfort, information, and emotional support. They do not provide medical care, so a doula at a home birth would be working in tandem with a midwife. The doula is looking out for you and your partner and can also help with small errands (like getting food or warm towels) and after-birth cleaning. At my home birth, I had a doula. She was an important extra set of hands for whatever was needed.

Many participants in the BornClear course choose to have home births. Interestingly enough, quite a few women who thought they wanted to have a hospital birth reconsidered this decision after taking the course and eventually chose childbirth in either a birthing center or at home. Again, there is no right or wrong answer here. All you need to focus on is making a decision that is consistent with all you want for yourself, your family, your baby.

— My Home Birth Story—

I knew that I wanted to give birth at home. I know myself, and I'm just not able to relax in a hospital. So I interviewed midwives, and when I met Roberta, we connected right away. She was intensely smart—intellectually, medically, emotionally, and spiritually. I asked her many questions and learned about her philosophy, her understanding of me, her experience, the equipment she brought, her strengths and weaknesses, and the beautiful stories about all of the women and the babies she had been with. To me, Roberta seemed truly divine. Once I knew we were going to work together, we were connected as a team.

I also created a back-up plan with a great doctor who had worked with Roberta. When I met with him, I asked him about his philosophy and how he worked. It was fascinating. He had mastered the surgical technique of doing a C-section and sewing the various layers of tissue so that the woman would heal quickly with the least amount of scar tissue and have the ability to deliver vaginally with much less risk for her next child. I learned that his wife, also a doctor, had birthed their children at home. After a long conversation in which I reviewed the options and the procedures, I felt safe with him. He was so funny. He said, "Now that we have met, you trust yourself, and we will never have to see each other again!"

At home, I was able to create the environment I knew would make me feel relaxed, which included certain foods and music. Each of my children's births was magical and beautiful. I was so proud of myself for all that I created for myself and my children. I videotaped their births and they watch their birth videos, truly witnessing their "birth days," on their birthdays each year. You can watch these videos on the BornClear Web site at www.BornClear.com.

Water Births (in a Hospital, in a Birthing Center, or at Home)

Water covers two-thirds of our planet, constitutes 78 percent of the human body at birth, and is probably the most significant element for life on Earth. Intuitively, human beings have always been drawn to the soothing, relaxing comfort of water. As Jessica Johnson and Dr. Michel Odent express in their beautiful book *We Are All Water Babies*, "Human beings have to live with 'two brains': the old, primitive, emotional brain on the one hand, and the new brain, the highly developed neocortex on the other hand. The neocortex has the power to inhibit or repress the instinctive brain in a great variety of situations, such as swimming, or giving birth, or any episode of sexual life. Water is the primary mediator or harmonizing agent in the relationship between our two brains."

Many women, midwives, and doctors acknowledge the analgesic effects of water during labor and birth, as well as the value of water in pain management. In almost any birthing setting, hot showers and hot towels are used to ease lower-back pain during contractions, hot compresses are applied to the perineum to help it to soften and stretch, and cool cloths are laid across the back of the neck and on the forehead to soothe and relax. When a woman in labor relaxes in a deep warm bath, free from gravity's pull on her body, and with sensory stimulation reduced, her body is less likely to release the catecholamines, the stress-related hormones. At the same time, the water can allow her body to produce pain inhibitors such as endorphins. This is the same mind-body recipe we've been talking about and will continue to discuss throughout this book.

Thousands of mothers who have experienced water births, including me, state that they would never consider laboring without water again. Water helps some women reach a state of consciousness in which their fear and resistance are diminished or removed completely. Many birthing women reported being better able to concentrate, focus, and go inward once they got into a tub of water. Doctors and midwives who attend water births find that the mere sound of water helps some women release their inhibitions.

Water will also help soften the tissues of the perineum, reducing the incidence and severity of tearing and eliminating the need for episiotomies. Dr. Michel Odent, a French physician and a proponent of water birth, reported that in one hundred water births he had attended, no episiotomies were performed and there were only twenty-nine cases of tearing, all of which were minor surface tears.

It is also thought that the ease of the mother who labors and gives birth in water is transferred to the child who is born in the water. And because the mother is more relaxed during this type of birth, she can be more emotionally available to immediately receive and become attached to her child. A baby's limbs can also unfold with greater ease during his or her first moments. Water softens the sensory overload that can be a part of birth. Lights and sounds are softer when perceived from under the water, and even the touch of the mother's skin is softened.

Water births encompass a range of practices. Besides a mother laboring and/or birthing in a tub, Dr. Frederick Leboyer introduced the idea of giving babies a warm bath immediately after birth. The Leboyer method places the infant into a basin of water heated to body temperature. The baby then experiences the comforting return to the sensations of the womb. During Leboyer baths, babies are often wide-eyed and attentive and smile as they move their arms and legs playfully in the water. They can even swim and propel themselves in the water.

It has been said that doctors and nurses can tell which babies have been born in water because they seem to act like little grown-ups. When I had my two children in water, this was my experience as well. Aside from the depth of comfort, warmth, and ease I felt while birthing in water, I was amazed when both of my children looked at me very clearly and consciously from under the water while coming to the surface. They were beautifully alert, and we were able to connect right away, visually and emotionally. A few days after the birth of my first child, Savannah, I took her out to a coffee shop for my first coffee in a while—espresso, thank goodness—and a woman sitting with her mother at the table next to us came over and asked me whether Savannah had been born in water. I was so surprised by this question, especially coming from a stranger. I answered yes and asked her how she knew. The woman smiled and said, "I can just tell. My daughter was born in water, too, so alert and clear."

The baby doesn't need to immediately breathe with his lungs during a water birth because he is still getting oxygen from the mother via the umbilical cord attached to the placenta. He doesn't start to breathe on his own until he reaches the open air, which stimulates the breathing reflex. After the baby is born, it is best to bring him to the surface as quickly and gently as possible. This is to avoid any problems if the placenta separates early.

Practitioners of water birth will scrupulously maintain a clean tub, so that the mother is not at risk of getting an infection from the water. It is commonly believed that the mother's own bacteria and blood pose no risk for the baby. In truth, it is important for the baby to become colonized with the mother's bacteria, which offers him some protection and can help develop his immune system.

The option of water birth can be used at home, in various birthing centers, and in some hospitals. More than 250 hospitals in the United States have successful water-birth programs, and some hospitals will allow you to bring your own rented pool as well. For more information on water births, including Waterbirth International, see the Resources section at the end of the book.

Putting It All Together

You should research each of these choices further and speak with various practitioners in your area, as well as with some of their previous patients/clients. The Resources section at the end of the book is an invaluable tool for strengthening your context. Discuss your decisions with your partner, and make sure that you are both on the same page.

Even if the two of you are completely aligned, be willing to reconsider your choice, given what you began to create for yourselves and your baby. Mentally "recheck" the choice you already made, and make sure that it really works for you. This choice should make you feel good; the decision should sit right with you. If specific thoughts or concerns crop up about the choice you made, make a list of those concerns, and see whether you can address each of them.

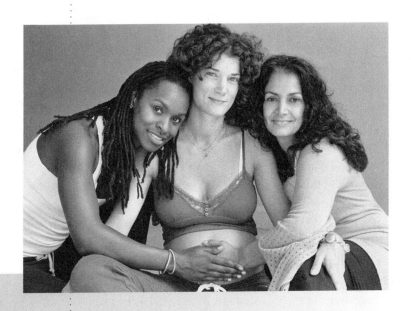

4 The BornClear Toolbox

T he BornClear toolbox combines many relaxation methods that you can use throughout your pregnancy and during childbirth. A lot of these methods fully integrate the mind and the body, teaching you a variety of ways that you can connect with your body—and your baby. Mastering these tools gives you the ability to temporarily shut out life's distractions and truly listen, hearing and feeling yourself and your baby at the deepest levels.

These exercises include visualizations, meditations, affirmations, writing exercises, art exercises, breathing techniques, hands-on work, physical exercises, personal growth exercises, and other methods and suggestions. The toolbox allows you to experiment with all of the possible ways you can integrate whatever you create into your childbirth, by trusting yourself and connecting with your baby.

The best way to use the toolbox is to read through the entire chapter first, then go back and see which exercises resonate with you. You will create a simple daily practice for each week that focuses on these exercises. Feel free to change your practices weekly. It's like picking a perfect meal from a Chinese food restaurant's menu, where you can choose whatever you desire. Follow as many suggestions as you are comfortable with, and put together a program that best fits your context. You are developing your own formula for success.

Have fun with all of these suggestions, and feel free to incorporate your family or friends into your practice. For example, on special evenings you and your partner can practice visualizations, take a soothing aromatherapy bath, or even have some quiet time while you walk together. The tools can be integrated into your life anywhere and everywhere. The key is to make sure that you use at least one of the tools every day, even if it is for a short time.

You will work with the BornClear tools throughout your pregnancy and during your birthing journey. They will also be available to you for the rest of your life as part of a healthy practice. You won't know in advance which tools you may want to use in the moment, however, so it's best if you are familiar with all of them. Practicing allows you to have access to these tools, which can make an enormous difference in bringing you closer—mentally, emotionally, physically, and spiritually—to anything you deal with during pregnancy and birth. Practicing these techniques reinforces your ability to relax as much as possible on "command." Just by thinking and wanting to feel relaxed, you will become relaxed. You'll learn to recognize this feeling of relaxation. This is exactly the "space of birth" that you need to be in, where there is less thinking and more feeling.

The Toolbox and the Mind-Body Connection

Your state of mind directly impacts how you feel, and how you feel can be influenced if you align your heart, body, and mind in the present moment. Your body's responses shift and change from instant to instant, in response to your train of thought and associated emotions. If you want to physically or emotionally "feel better," you have to take actions that best support the outcome you want.

During these practices, you will experience a feeling of going inward, within yourself. You will actually learn how to create a calm and relaxing environment in which you produce additional endorphins in your body. At a mental level, you are learning to trust yourself and your body. The more you practice, the quieter you will become and the easier and more automatic the mind-body connection will be. You may feel that you have tapped more deeply into yourself and are more connected to the baby. This is when you will really start to trust yourself.

You are closer to the space of birth than you realize. Tap into your personalized divinity by picking various methods in the toolbox that already resonate with you. Build on the memories that you have to create a safe and deep space. It could be five minutes every day of sitting quietly or five minutes of Ujjayi breathing. You might join a weekly prenatal yoga class or get regular prenatal massages or even acupuncture. Maybe you will listen to your favorite music or light candles. All of these tools will help you create alone, quiet, inward time.

As you practice, you will learn to slow down. Your daily life right now may not be about connecting; you may feel that you are trying your best, but all that you manage to do is get through what is on your plate. I want you to slow the pace of your life during this pregnancy so that you can feel what is going on around and within you.

Later, after your baby is born, you can continue to use these tools any time in your life: while breast-feeding, during a stressful situation, whenever you are upset, when you find yourself complaining, when you are trying to create or to manifest something, when you are searching for a deeper understanding of yourself, when you can't sleep, when you feel anxious, and when you try to calm your children. This is really a toolbox for life.

Every month, you can increase the amount of time you spend on whatever practices you choose. By the eighth and the ninth months, you should be devoting up to an hour daily to yourself and your baby, enjoying the last days of this journey as much as you can. Following are my suggestions for incorporating the toolbox into your life, but feel free to use it more often as needed.

- Months 1–3: Practice three times a week for a minimum of fifteen minutes each time.

- Months 4–7: Practice five times a week for a minimum of twenty minutes each time. You can break these up into ten minutes twice a day if that is better for your schedule. Try to integrate at least one, possibly two, prenatal yoga classes a week into your life.

- Month 8: Begin to nurture yourself even more. A daily practice for a minimum of fifteen minutes and two prenatal yoga classes a week are in order. If you can, take in a prenatal massage twice this month.

- Month 9: Do a daily practice twice a day for twenty minutes each time. If you feel up to it, attend at least one prenatal yoga class weekly and one prenatal massage; these are not included in the time allotted for your daily practices.

BornClear Breathing

The following breathing methods can be used throughout your pregnancy and during childbirth. Learning yogic breathing can help you bring consciousness to the breathing process, achieve mastery of your mind and listen to what is going on inside your head. Training your brain to do one thing at a time promotes an ability to focus.

Experiment with all of these techniques: some will make you feel more relaxed, others will give you greater focus and will even increase your energy levels. Some breathing methods will be used in later exercises, so it is important to be familiar with all of them.

Many of these exercises are based on yogic breathing techniques. In yoga, it is believed that control of the prana, or life force, leads to control of the mind. Breathing exercises are called *pranayamas,* which means "to control the prana."

Before you begin any breathing practice, find a quiet, clean, and peaceful space in which to work. Take a comfortable seated position and properly align your spine as straight as possible.

Ujjayi (victorious) breathing. Ujjayi breathing involves taking full complete breaths, inhaling and exhaling, through the nose. While breathing in and out through your nose, your mouth should remain closed. The incoming air makes a soft hissing noise on the back of your throat. On the exhalation, move the breath downward by constricting your throat muscles so that you make the sound of the ocean. This technique enables your body to actually warm up. You are getting maximum energy and heat from your breaths. With each exhalation, try to breathe out the tension and stress you were keeping within your body.

Gentle belly breathing. Many expectant women experience a sense of breathlessness during pregnancy. Belly breathing will allow you to relax and regain your breath. In this exercise, you will learn how to move breath up from your belly instead of through your chest. This exercise will open the belly and allow the diaphragm to move deeper into your abdomen on the inhalation and farther up to squeeze your lungs and support your heart on the exhalation. This breathing practice will not hurt or affect your baby in any way.

To do this exercise, lie down on your back on a bed, a yoga mat, or even a carpeted floor. Place your hands (one on top of the other) on your belly, with the center of your lower hand touching your navel. Focus your breath so that your belly expands as you inhale and retracts as you exhale. If your belly seems tight, lightly massage the outside edge of your belly button. Notice how your belly begins to soften and relax. If your belly does not move as you breathe, press down with your hands on your belly as you exhale. Then as you inhale, gradually release the tension. Try this several times. Notice how your belly begins to open more on the inhalation.

Although it's easiest if you are lying down, you can also practice belly breathing while you are sitting, standing, or even walking. It is an excellent practice to try before you get out of bed in the morning or if you have difficulty falling asleep. It is also beneficial whenever you are anxious or tense. Belly breathing will be very useful during contractions, when you are looking for a way to relax and find stamina during labor. I also practice this exercise with my children when they feel anxious or have trouble going to sleep.

Viloma breathing. Viloma means "against the natural flow." In Viloma breathing, the inhalations and the exhalations are interrupted with brief pauses. Viloma supports the nervous system and brings a sense of tranquility to the mind. It encourages the balance of the upward and downward flow of energy.

To do this exercise, find a comfortable seated position. Gently exhale all of the air from your lungs. Inhale through both nostrils. On the exhalation, stop when the air is halfway out. Control the air as it leaves your lungs through the nostrils. Make the outflow of air even on both sides. Hold your breath for about four seconds before continuing to exhale all of the air out of your lungs. Do this practice for at least five to ten breaths each time.

Birth cycle breathing. This is a great exercise to build resilience in the birth canal, bring awareness to the pelvic floor muscles, and practice "bearing down." The downward flow of energy is important to connect with during pregnancy because this rhythm will become pronounced during your labor. This type of breathing works well with guided visualizations and can be practiced in a squatting position.

To do this exercise, inhale through your nose, engaging and lifting your pelvic floor as you deeply breathe in. Feel your energy down through your solar plexus. Send your breath into your belly, down and out through the birth canal, and into the earth. Then exhale through your nose.

Rhythmic breathing. This exercise is timed to the rhythm of your heartbeat. Inhalations and exhalations should be done to the same number of beats, as this establishes an even rhythm. Do this exercise three times the first week and add one more round each week, until you are doing seven complete breaths.

To do this exercise, get into an easy cross-legged position on the floor or a yoga mat, or sit on a well-supported chair. Keep your spine straight, with your hands on your knees, and start by taking a few deep breaths. Place the second, third, and fourth fingers of your right hand on your left wrist to find your pulse. Carefully feel your pulse beat, and after a short while start counting in your head four pulses. Continue to mentally count from one to four until you fall into this rhythm and can follow it without holding your pulse. Then put your hands on your knees and take a deep breath while counting from one to four; hold your breath while counting from one to two; exhale while again counting from one to four. Next, exhale slowly for eight seconds. For the first six seconds allow your collar bone, chest, and ribs to relax, so that your breath goes out automatically. For the last two seconds, push your stomach in gently, to expel all of the air from your lungs. Keep your stomach in this position for four seconds before you take the next breath.

Walking breathing. This exercise is done in exactly the same way as rhythmic breathing, except that you do it while walking. Use each step as a count, similar to the pulse beat used in rhythmic breathing.

To do this exercise, stand erect, exhale first, and then start walking, with your right foot first. Take four steps while inhaling, hold your breath in for two steps, exhale for four steps, and hold your breath out for two steps. Without stopping, continue the routine: inhale on four steps, hold your breath in for two steps, and so forth. Do not interrupt the walking—keep it rhythmic. The breathing should be done in one continuous flow: inhale one deep breath to the count of four, hold it to the count of two, exhale to the count of four, and again hold the emptiness to the count of two. This completes one round. Do five such rounds each time you attempt this exercise.

Alternate nostril breathing. This exercise will clean and rejuvenate your vital channels of energy. During this exercise, you will breathe through only one nostril at a time. This exercise produces optimal function in both sides of the brain, enhancing creativity and logical, verbal activity. This also creates a more balanced person, since both halves of the brain are functioning properly. Yogis consider this to be the best technique to calm the mind and the nervous system.

To do this exercise, close your right nostril with your right thumb and inhale through the left nostril. Do this to the count of four seconds. Immediately close the left nostril with your right ring finger and little finger, and at the same time remove your thumb from the right nostril, and exhale through this nostril. Do this to the count of eight seconds. This completes a half round. Inhale through your right nostril to the count of four seconds. Close the right nostril with your right thumb, remove your right ring finger and little finger from the left nostril, and exhale through the left nostril to the count of eight seconds. This completes one full round.

Start by doing three rounds, and add one per week until you are doing seven rounds. Alternate nostril breathing should not be practiced if you have a cold or if your nasal passages are blocked.

Taoist relaxation yoga breathing. Taoist yoga is especially good for relaxation and to remove anxiety. It gives prompt, quick, and temporary relief. The method is very simple: "Listen to your breathing." Nothing more is needed, except persistence and patience in listening. If you do not persist, your attention will stray back into anxieties. When you attend to your breathing, you tend to take deeper, longer breaths and, in the process, quiet your mental activities as your mind harmonizes itself with the slower, and slowing, rhythm of the breathing. By listening, you must focus your attention on the sound of your breaths, thereby withdrawing it from whatever has been disturbing, exciting, and fatiguing your mind.

Visualizations

Visualization is an ancient practice that combines mentally creating images, relaxing, and meditating. My visualizations are inspired by many sources, including the classic book *Creative Visualization* by Shakti Gawain. Visualization is one of the many BornClear tools that allow you to reach deep levels of relaxation, master going inward, and drop deeply into yourself, quickly and easily. This mastery will help you shut out the distractions in your life and truly listen, hearing and feeling yourself and your baby at the deepest levels. At the same time that you are relaxing, you release the body's most powerful pain reducer, endorphins.

To begin each of the following visualizations, find a room where you can practice without distractions. Sit down in a comfortable position, or lie down on the floor or another supportive surface. Read through all of the instructions beforehand so that you are comfortable with them. Or have someone else, such as your spouse or partner, read these instructions to you. He or she should read them slowly and in a relaxing voice, infusing peace into the words. The activity of reading should be calming for the reader, as well as for you.

Begin each visualization with the following full body relaxation exercise:

Take five Ujjayi breaths, breathing in deeply with your mouth closed. As you breathe in, take in calmness and ease, and as you breathe out, release all of the day's tensions, all aches, all thoughts, all heaviness, let it all leave. With each breath you are taking in all that you want to relax and letting go of all that you want to release—conversations from the day, things to do, time, all of it . . . let it go. After three full breaths, feel the heaviness of your eyelids and begin to slowly close your eyes. Drop your shoulders, planting your weight into the earth. Relax your whole body, and let calmness flow from the crown of your head and move to your forehead, your eyes, your cheekbones, your jaw—let it fall toward your stomach, surrounding your baby, your lower back, your hips, your upper legs, the backs of your legs, your knees, shins, calves, ankles, heels, feet, toes, let it all go and bathe yourself in full relaxation, quieting your mind and body, all the while getting heavier and quieter.

If it is easier to visualize a relaxing fluid that moves into every part of your body, give it your favorite color and bathe each part of yourself with peacefulness.

Your private place visualization. Bring your mind to all of the places you have ever been where you felt peaceful and safe. It could be your home, a special room, the ocean, a meadow, swimming under the ocean, the mountains, a favorite vacation, or even a memory. Bring yourself there with your mind's eye. Feel it fully, and notice how you feel. Look around—notice the visual details, see whether anyone is with you who completes your feelings of safety and peacefulness. Smell the air, and notice whether it is day or night. Soak it all in and feel yourself there. Let yourself really enjoy this private sanctuary that is all yours. Know that you can drop into this private sanctuary whenever you want to—this visualization is now associated with calmness, and it is all created by you.

Once you can really be in this place, bring your context and all that you have created with your partner about your birth, how you want it to feel, how you want to feel, and see yourself holding your newborn baby in this place. Visualize it surrounded by a balloon or a bubble of your favorite color. I like gold. Now send the balloon off into the "air" and share with the universe your private sanctuary, with all of your intentions, visions, wishes, and blessings to be manifested. Let it go.

As you bring this vision or visualization to a close, take a few final Ujjayi breaths, and bring life back into all of the places in your body, move your hands, wiggle your toes, and when you are ready and only when you are ready, slowly and gently open your eyes. Know that your private sanctuary is here for you always.

"Talk with your body" affirmation. You can talk to your body just as you would talk to a friend. When you talk to yourself or your body, you are moving into the awareness that you are not only your mind or your body but one whole. This is empowering and can help reduce stress or anxiety, a state of mind that depletes you, rather than energizing you. I believe that discomfort or disease happens when there is an imbalance of some kind, so when you put your heart, body, and mind back in harmony (aligned with the breath), you feel more peaceful and your vital energy begins to rise up. But you have to start the process by commanding this shift to happen.

You can do this simple and effective exercise while you are moving (walking, biking, and so forth) or in seated meditation. Start with a minute of deep, regular, even breaths until you feel yourself becoming centered and calm. Then feel yourself breathe into your body, focusing on one specific part, like your feet. Repeat out loud or mentally to yourself, "Thank you, I love you." Repeat these phrases to every part of your body, passing on your love and gratitude, no matter what state your body part is in. Then for another couple of minutes repeat aloud or mentally, "Body, now restore yourself to a state of perfect health. I accept and expect the best."

Then do . . . expect the best.

Regenerating yourself visualization. Visualize a large tube inside of you that stands upright, stretching from your head to your toes. This tube is flexible. Fill it with fluid of any color that you love. This beautiful, soothing fluid contains deep relaxation and endorphins. Imagine pouring the contents of the tube into the top of your head—it will eventually fill your entire body. Begin pouring slowly, filling your feet, moving up your legs, into your knees and thighs, your hips and pelvis, all around your belly and baby, into your upper chest and neck, throughout your back and into your arms and hands, and within your face to the top of your head. At any point in time if you feel tension in your body, bring this soothing fluid to that area. Bathe in this fluid, and wash away the tension or negative sensations. During birth, you can bring this fluid of deep relaxation and endorphins to any area of your body that you choose. Use any color that works for you.

The "pink bubble" visualization. This exercise is very soothing and you can do it anywhere. I have chosen the color pink, which resonates with love and the heart, like the color of rose quartz, but you can create your bubble in any color you wish.

Imagine something that you want to happen: it could be the context you created for your birthing experience, it could be you and your partner and your new baby, anything you want to manifest. Imagine that it has already happened. Picture it clearly in your mind—see it, feel it, sense it. Now surround your vision with a pink bubble. This bubble holds your heart's desire and resonates with what is in perfect harmony with your essence, your spirit.

Let go of the bubble and imagine it floating off into the universe, the sky, and the clouds. This symbolizes your trust in letting it go, knowing, believing, trusting that it will come to you, come into existence.

Water goddess visualization. Imagine yourself as the fertile sea. The sea gives and supports life: every mineral that exists on the planet can be found in the healing waters of the sea. The womb is an abundant and powerful space, with its own rhythm that moves in sync with the cosmos. It has all that it needs to develop and sustain new life. Your womb is the ocean that supports life thriving within. You are abundant, full of water, full of life. As the ocean inhales, the tide pulls back, and sand, seashells, and seaweeds are revealed. As the ocean exhales, the tide rolls back in, splashing the shore. If you pick up a shell, you will find that same echo of breath from the ocean, audible inside the seashell. When you listen to your belly, you hear a beautiful sound of a tiny heartbeat within your fertile waters. Imitate the sound that the ocean makes when you breathe with your Ujjayi breath.

Mother Tree visualization. This visualization combines with movement. To begin, follow the relaxation piece found at the beginning of this section until you are completely relaxed. Then, stand up as you focus on the following text:

> Women are like trees: grounded, purposeful, and bearers of new life. A tree is so balanced because it is working in concert with two forces—gravity and levity. While the tree is rooting herself firmly into the soil, sending roots deeper into the earth, she is simultaneously reaching with her branches toward the heavens. We also are grounded during pregnancy. We experience the sensation of gravity as our bodies become larger. At the same time there is a strong levitational force at work. This force is working to raise us toward the heavens as much as we are being pulled through our feet toward the earth. Keep your balance between both spaces. As you're being pulled toward

the earth, lift through your spine, engage your pelvic floor, and lower your abdominal muscles. To ground yourself, stand firm, both feet gripping the earth with your toes.

Using colors: A visualization inspired by the chakras. We each have a natural response to certain colors. You already are sensitive and in tune to color, some colors more than others. Notice how colors make you feel. Certain colors make you feel light, like the color of a brilliant blue sky. Other colors reflect your current mood. What color did you choose to wear today? What is the color of your favorite, most memorable sunset? What are the colors in your home? This exercise will teach you how to use color as a tool to relax, trust, and feel yourself. Each time you practice this relaxation, you will be able to go deeper and deeper into a state of being that you will use in labor. Have your partner record this exercise for you, so that you can listen to it any time, including in the bath. Once you have practiced with your partner and/or listened to a taping, you will be able to create the flow of the visualization for yourself, quietly in your mind.

All of the colors are beautiful tools. They can be called on at any point during the birth. You can choose a particular color or colors for whatever you may be dealing with in the moment: to help soothe the sensation of pain and make it subside, to calm your whole body, to tap into your ability to trust yourself, to make you remember all that you have created for your childbirth, or to become connected with your baby and work as a unified team.

You can personalize this exercise by integrating the color or colors that resonate with you most. Bring those colors to the various areas of your body where you might feel pain or need support: your lower pelvis, your lower and middle abdomen, your lower and middle back, your upper abdomen, your heart, your upper back, your throat, the space between your eyes, the back or the top of your head. Color yourself entirely, including the space around you and through you.

The exercise begins as you feel calmness filtering through your body. Your baby inside you is growing and developing beautifully.

With each breath that passes, you are growing in confidence and assurance that your baby's entrance into this world will be a beautiful, joyous event. Birthing is a natural process. Your body, your mind, and your baby will all be working in complete natural harmony to accomplish this wondrous event. These thoughts relax you as you go deeper and deeper into calmness and peace.

Once you are fully relaxed and breathing naturally, bring your mind to the color red. Let yourself resonate with the relaxing feeling of the color red, feel how big it is—picture a soft, red blanket that you will lie on. Imagine the shade of red that best soothes you—is it a juicy red strawberry, a rich red nail polish? Pick your favorite red, and as you lie on this thick lush blanket of red, continue to see this color down around the lower part of your body, around your pelvis, infusing a gentle flow of "your" red all the way down to your feet, starting at your upper legs, and flowing down to your lower legs, your calves, your ankles, your feet, and your toes—all relaxing into your lush, very soft blanket of red.

Now picture the color orange, the shade of orange that most resonates with you: your favorite sunset, a bowl of beautiful plump juicy oranges, small pumpkins, the orange leaves of fall. Use the warmth of this orange color to release any tensions in and around your lower and middle abdomen and around your child. This warmth is exactly at the temperature you love most. It is the perfect warmth of orange. Breathe in this warmth, and use your orange in any way you want to.

Move on to yellow—the feeling and color of sunlight, honey, a yellow gold, your favorite yellow crayon, a bed of yellow rose petals or orchids—and bathe yourself in an ocean of beautiful yellow. Immerse yourself in this feeling of yellow, feeling it flow through you and around you. Releasing, relaxing, feeling deeply calm in the yellow and all that you bring to it. . . . Take your time.

Next comes green, the most lush soft green grass, a bowl of green limes, the green of the mountains, green leaves on trees, the power and beauty of green in nature—feel this green. It is so soothing, so earthy. Feel the air of green all around you, and bring this color of soothing green to your heart. You are relaxing, infused with the comforting color green, and it allows you to trust yourself and fall deeply onto this cozy blanket of green.

Now feel the color blue, the brightest, most beautiful blue sky you have ever seen. Wrap yourself and your baby in this comforting feeling of blue. Feel the peace, the serenity of your blue. Send this color in and around your baby, with both of you feeling total ease and peace, trusting life, nature, and yourselves fully. Bring this blue around your neck in the front and the back, releasing all thoughts about what you need to communicate and what you have not communicated. Feel free in the blue air that you are gliding on, walking within, and surrounding yourself in.

Think of lavender, this beautiful mix of blue, red, and white. Create a pillow of lavender to rest your head and your entire body on, falling heavily onto your lavender body pillow of support and comfort. Let all of your worries, thoughts, and tensions seep out of your body and your mind, and let your body fall heavily and be supported by the lavender. Bring the lavender between your eyes and see all that you have been creating for your baby to come: the birth, your partner, yourself, the beauty of all that you are doing now, mothering yourself in lavender.

The last color is white; think about the purifying freedom that comes with your white. Bring your thoughts of white to the top of your head, surrounding yourself in a bubble of white. Release any negative thoughts out of the top of your head through the bubble of white. All that surrounds you in this nurturing white bubble is you knowing yourself, your essence, the beauty of who you are, the beauty of all you are creating, the beauty of this new person coming into your life. Trust your own internal wisdom, use your white.

Transforming pain or anxiety into an object visualization. Many of us experience sensations that we regard as unpleasant: tension, stress, strain, and discomfort. There is an image that can bring you peace, comfort, contentment, and relief—deep relaxation. This is another method that is so powerful, it can remove all of your symptoms of stress and strain. I know that stress is a very subjective feeling, so I have created a way to channel your unpleasant sensations into an object.

When you experience pain or discomfort or if you feel tense or anxious, you will take that unwanted feeling and give it a shape. Allow yourself to visualize that shape. It can be any kind of shape: it can be an object or a geometric design. It can be soft, and it can be in a certain color. Whatever shape or object first comes into your mind is the right shape for you; don't try to force the shape, just let it happen. As you go deeper, feel that you are peaceful, calm, and very relaxed.

Now, imagine the size of the shape. You begin to realize that the shape is a symbol of your discomfort, and the larger the shape is, the more severe the discomfort feels. The smaller the shape is, the less the discomfort you feel. See whether you can make the shape larger, and then make it smaller. See whether it is easier to make the shape bigger or smaller. If you have difficulty making the shape smaller, use a few tricks. If the shape is a balloon, you can make a small hole in it with a fine needle, or you can kick it away so that it is swept into the atmosphere. You can put it on a boat or an airplane or tie it to the back of a train and let it drift away, out over the landscape of your mind.

Next we'll change the color of your object. First choose a color that is bright and vivid. Let the color fade until it is just barely visible. As you make the object smaller, take the color out of it. Every time you do this, you'll find that you can do it more and more effortlessly, until the pain or the upset is completely clear and then gone.

Meditation

Meditation is one way you can give yourself personal attention. It helps the body and the mind rest, relax, and rejuvenate and has many health benefits as well. Studies have shown that daily meditation can help people overcome anxiety and depression and can deepen their concentration, stimulate their creativity, and lower blood pressure. It is an easy practice that will help you calm down quickly, which is why it is a perfect birthing tool.

Meditation can also be a spiritual practice. Many people experience meditation as a form of prayer, where their divinity "speaks" to them, rather than just listening. Others experience "guidance" or inner wisdom when the mind is quiet, and they meditate for this purpose. You can meditate on a single question until an answer comes (although some people would say that this engages your thinking mind too much), or you can meditate to clear your mind and accept whatever is given to you.

You can use a variety of techniques to tap into this state, and I've listed some of my favorites here. You can meditate wherever you are, even if you are able to steal only five minutes from your busy day. Sit comfortably and quietly with your eyes closed, breathe fully, and let your thoughts go. Meditation is a gift, not a chore, so enjoy it and make it simple for yourself so that you will do it.

Basic meditation technique. Sit in a comfortable position or lie down. Quiet your mind by thinking of nothing. It's not always easy to do this, so don't be ashamed if you have to practice only this part at first. One good way to begin is to think of yourself as an "observer of your thoughts," merely noticing what the narrative voice in your head says but not engaging it. As thoughts materialize in your mind, just let them go.

Focused meditation. This technique has you focus on something intently but without engaging your thoughts about it. You can focus on something visually, such as a statue or a candle flame; something auditory, like a metronome or a tape of ocean waves; or something constant—for example, your breath. Stay in the present moment and circumvent the constant stream of commentary from your conscious mind, allowing yourself to slip into an altered state of consciousness.

Activity-oriented meditation. With this type of meditation, you engage in a repetitive "mindless" activity, such as gardening, creating artwork, or practicing yoga. Each of these activities allows you to get "in a zone" and experience "flow" as you accomplish your task without really thinking.

Mindfulness techniques. Mindfulness can be a form of meditation that, like activity-oriented meditation, doesn't really *look* like meditation. It involves staying in the present moment, rather than thinking about the future or the past. (Again, this is more difficult than it seems.) Focusing on sensations you feel in your body is one way to stay "in the now"; focusing on emotions and where you feel them in your body (not *examining why* you feel them, but just *experiencing them* as sensations) is another way.

BornClear heart meditation. Nikki Costello, a yoga and meditation teacher, created this heart meditation for BornClear. In it, we strive to create a space inside the chest to acknowledge a heart big enough and strong enough to support a new life. This gives us the courage to recognize our immense capacity to love.

Choose a comfortable seat—it can be a chair or the floor. If you are in a chair, place your feet firmly on the ground. Settle into your hips and legs. Allow your spine to gently elongate upward while you rest your hands on your thighs. With a deep inhalation, lift the sides of your chest and your sternum upward. As you exhale, draw your shoulders back behind your chest and gather the support of your shoulder blades on your back. Each time you inhale, allow your breath to rise and spread into the region of your heart. Each time you exhale, stay present to the sensation of the breath going out as your chest remains lifted, open, and calm. Stay here, infusing your heart center with the fullness and ease of steady, rhythmic breaths.

Keep your eyes open for a few minutes. Learn to keep your posture alert and focused as you direct your attention to the movement of your breath inside your chest. Allow your ribcage to become wider on the sides, full in the back, and lifted in the front. Once you are able to be still and maintain a good posture, you are ready to close your eyes. Relax the skin on your forehead and let your eyelids close from top to bottom. Relax your cheeks, lips, tongue, and jaws. Allow the expression on your face to be neutral and serene. With your eyes closed, direct your gaze downward toward the heart. Continue to follow the movement of your breath.

As you sit for meditation, let everything drop into your heart. All of your thoughts—let them drop there. All of your emotions— let them be there. Now, focus on the following:

Your heart is big enough and strong enough to contain every- thing. Each inhalation is a reminder to be full and complete because the container of your chest is supporting you. And each exhalation allows you to soften and rest inside the space of the heart. In this way, each moment is a birth and death, like the in breath and the out breath. Each time you remember to lift and open your chest, the heart gets bigger and stronger.

When you come out of the meditation, reflect on what you experienced. You can record your feelings or insights, or choose to hold them in your memory.

Owning a Mantra

The idea behind using a mantra is to repeat a phrase that helps you focus and go inward, instantly. Choose any mantra that speaks to you—it could be a sentence from your favorite novel, letters of the alphabet, numbers, a word, names, or a phrase. I am connected to the phrase "Om Namah Shivaya," which is Sanskrit for "I honor the divinity that lies within me," and that is my mantra. Feel free to try mine, or another one that I love is the great mantra of Buddhism, "Om Mani Padme Hum"("Hail to the jewel in the lotus.") *Om,* as we said, was the hidden aspect of God. *Mani padme* is the Radiant Jewel (*mani*) in the Lotus (*padme*). It expresses the enlightened mind, the mind as it rises up to the surface of illumination.

To use your mantra, take a handful of deep cleansing breaths and begin to repeat your mantra in a natural, rhythmic way. For example, if your mantra is the counting numbers, you would say, "111, 222, 333, 444 . . ."

Some women like to take their mantras into the delivery room to use when they are in labor. One of my clients told me that she spent five hours of her labor simply chanting, "Let go." This helped her breathe, focus, and relinquish herself to the birth.

Writing Exercises

The following writing exercises can help you relax during your pregnancy. They are a useful aid when you create your context, and they also promote positive feelings. Use your free time to write to support your goals for achieving clarity and personal growth. Although you can't practice writing exercises during childbirth, they will help you prepare your thoughts for your journey.

Writing affirmations. Sometimes we need reminders. I know for myself that reminders can bring me back to the present if I am moving too fast or I feel overwhelmed. Affirmations are these types of reminders. They are positive statements that describe a desired situation and that you repeat many times to impress the subconscious mind to trigger a positive action. Affirmations need to be said in the affirmative, with attention, conviction, interest, and desire. You can create any affirmation you want, starting with "I am." For example, "I am prepared for my baby to come."

This is a fun and very active creative exercise. Take any affirmation that resonates with you and write it out ten times in a row without stopping, really thinking about the words and the feeling of those words as you write them. Feel free to change the affirmation if you think of a better way to express this sentiment while you continue to write without stopping. When you are done, place these affirmations in various spots in your home as visual reminders. Stick one on your phone, on the bathroom mirror, on your desk, and by your bed. You can even record the affirmation and listen to it while driving, in the house, or in the bathtub.

Gratitude writing. Gratitude has the power to help shift your energy immediately. When you are immersed in fear, worry, anger, depression, or any negative state of mind, you need to reconnect with what you are thankful for.

Create a gratitude list of all the people and the aspects of your life that you are thankful for. Your list can include your family, your health, your body, your ability to walk, the sunset, a home, your partner, your baby, and so on. Be present to all that you are grateful for as you write the list. Feeling gratitude creates positive energy, which is also relaxing. You are focusing on all that is good versus on all that is wrong. This practice also keeps you "in the moment"—living in neither the past nor the future because gratitude is in the present.

First-thought writing. This exercise was inspired by a trip I took to Taos, New Mexico. I attended a writing workshop with Natalie Goldberg, the author of *Writing Down the Bones*. Natalie shared this technique as a way for you to get to what you are really feeling. It allows you to capture great honesty without an internal sensor. As you do this exercise, you will feel unencumbered by your ego—the mechanism in you that tries to control and rationalize your actions. This exercise is also a great way to release anxiety and fears or uncover what you are feeling, allowing you to be at peace, feel yourself, hear yourself, and fully know yourself.

You will need to time this exercise, so find a place to write where you can use a timer. Choose the time you will write: five minutes, ten, fifteen, it is up to you, and it can change every time you practice. Whatever amount of time you pick, you will write without stopping and without picking your pen off the paper until that amount of time has passed. All the while, you will be writing from your heart. You will not cross out or edit what you have written. Don't worry about spelling, grammar, or punctuation. This is stream-of-consciousness writing. Feel free to lose control. Don't think, don't get logical. If something comes up in your writing that is scary or naked, dive right into it and keep going. This kind of writing can stir up memories, emotions, and inspiration.

You can choose what you want to write about. Start by picking one single word and then write from there. For example, I once started with the word *cloud,* and so many feelings came up as I was writing, all of them flowing from my conscious, subconscious, and even unconscious mind. The exercise is very freeing and revealing.

You can use this exercise to help you develop the context for your childbirth or to create the conversations you need to have with your birth team. Use it to find ways to communicate with your baby—write to your baby, and see what shows up. You can write about creating and using the chemicals in your body—the endorphins, oxytocin. Write about trusting yourself, surrendering, your love for yourself, love for your partner, life as a new family . . . the subjects, as well as the possibilities, are limitless.

Keep a dream journal. Start to pay more attention to your dreams. One way to do this is by keeping a dream journal. This can help you explore what comes up from your subconscious. Connect it to everything you are working on in this book: your excitement, your fears, concerns, or things you still need to work out before the childbirth or in your life. You can even use dreams to get in touch with your baby. Many of my clients have told me that they communicated with their unborn babies through their dreams. Sometimes a name came to them for the baby, or they saw what the baby looked like.

I remember having a dream of Orion, my son, before he was born. In the dream he was laughing so joyfully, looking at me. This is exactly his spirit today!

Baby journal. Journaling is a powerful tool to deepen your understanding of new developments in your life. When you express feelings through an artistic process such as writing in a journal, their essence can be seen more clearly, and often the resulting awareness brings a sense of understanding, clarity, and freedom. In this dimension of creative expression, powerful ideas can arise freely. Fears and worries can be released, and new possibilities can be realized spontaneously.

There are a few elements that create a climate for powerful journaling. Commit to doing it every day. In the beginning, it makes a difference to also do it at the same time each day. You can easily set up your journaling spot, and each morning (or evening) gather your thoughts and sit with your journal and some art supplies (paints, markers, stickers, collage materials, stamps). Burn a candle and play some music that relaxes or inspires you. Let the pen do the writing, and enjoy the ride. Take a photograph every day or make a drawing or a painting, and describe what is interesting to you. Or, start by asking yourself a question. Then just let the words flow from you and from your child within.

This journal can be for you or for your baby, a beautiful ritual of creating a keepsake. It is another way to bond with your child now, as well as later in life. You can write to your baby in this journal, paint in it, paste photos from sonograms and daily life experiences, and record some of the adventures you have while you are pregnant.

I started these journals for both of my children. I began writing to them when I was pregnant. Reading the journals now is very moving for me. Sometimes my writing was very serious, and at other times it was very playful. I have kept up this ritual for years now. It is an incredible time capsule, and I enjoy going back to the journals with my children and sharing what I was experiencing, feeling, and seeing in that "real time" way.

Honesty log. A commitment to honesty always leads to peace and love, for yourself and for others.

The honesty log is something you can keep daily or weekly, however often feels right to you. Write down all of the ideas that you need to communicate in a notebook. They might be thoughts that you want to clarify for yourself or ideas or issues that you need to resolve with someone else. You can describe events or people whom you want to acknowledge to show proper appreciation. You can also write about things that bother or upset you. You may also want to recognize things that you have left unattended or "messy"— bills to pay, a conversation you never completed, or a book you never returned to a friend, even though you promised you would. The log can address whatever is currently on your mind.

When you read through this log, you can see which actions you need to take to feel at peace with yourself and with people in your life. This is a great exercise to do with your partner on a weekly or monthly basis to ensure that there is no buildup of assumptions, upsets, resentments, disappointment, hurt feelings, or misalignments. Later, you can continue this practice with your children, thereby taking an important step toward creating a completely clear and honest, open relationship with them.

Writing for healing exercise. We experience life every day; things happen to us, including incidents that compel us to make decisions unconsciously or consciously, or we make agreements with ourselves about our lives, other people, and ourselves. Some of these decisions form behaviors and habits that we are not proud of. This writing exercise will allow you to identify these agreements and come to terms with them, thereby returning to your true self.

On a blank piece of paper, you will create two lists. The first can be put together from any of the following possibilities: negative or painful memories, major or minor things that happened in your life that are still upsetting, and/or memorable conversations or experiences. Next to each of these aspects, see if you can determine what decision or agreement you have internally created that relates directly to them. For example, you may have a memory of your mother yelling at you when you were little, and after that experience you decided that you were "stupid."

Now that you recognize the connection between the event and the realization that followed it, you may be able to see the powerful impact that the event has had on your life. Take this opportunity to delve deeper into those experiences so that you can truly put them behind you. You could interview the people involved in your memory to see what they remember. Your perception of the event may not match theirs, and realizing that things did not occur as you have remembered them may allow you to bring clarity and closure to a deep misunderstanding.

Then, use the second list to keep track of when these same events or memories make you upset. Record your feelings as they arise, then see if you can undo the damage that is causing your negative feelings. The exercise will help you stop blaming other people or situations that upset you. It is a profound exercise that requires awareness, discipline, and patience.

For example, one time I had a conversation with my ex-husband that deeply upset me. I was so bothered by his words that it took me by surprise. Instead of responding immediately with anger, I excused myself and went to sit quietly under a tree until I could identify the feelings that surrounded my reaction. First, I had to get over my initial criticism of myself for leaving the "scene of the crime." Once I realized that removing myself from his presence was really the best idea, I could focus on the feelings I was experiencing. As I sat beneath the tree, four words popped into my head: "you are not loveable." I thought about those words and realized that my reaction to my ex-husband stemmed from an old wound that didn't involve him at all. I remembered that when I was very young, my relationship with my father had seemed distant. Even though he was a good man, he was not emotionally available. I remembered as a young girl expressing to him all of my passion and excitement and realizing that I did not get much back.

I realized that back in my past, I had formed a decision about my father based on how he had responded to me. As I sat under the tree, I was able to see it all, to identify what I had constructed for myself, and to understand how this agreement played out in all of my relationships. With clarity and focus, I said aloud, "This agreement is a lie. I am loving and completely loveable, and I will no longer allow this patter, this decision to live." In that moment, I abolished that agreement with myself and was crystal clear about the essence of who I am.

Therapeutic Art Exercises

Art can be expressive, relaxing, and revealing. Creating art in this way allows you to release feelings and thoughts nonverbally, which is very freeing.

You don't have to be talented to do this exercise: don't say no to the experience before you try it. Buy an unlined portfolio book in an art supply store so that you can keep all of your artwork in one place. Feel free to draw, paint, or sketch your images. You can create artwork for any aspect of your context, beginning with consciously conceiving and working all the way through delivery and birthing. This exercise should be fun and liberating, not tension-provoking. You can even get some of your friends and family members together and do this in a group.

When I was in labor with Savannah, I drew the way the contractions felt in her baby journal—it really showed me and the people on my birth team what I was experiencing. You can also use clay during birthing—squeezing and forming the clay can help you work through pressures, feelings, sensations, and pain.

Collage

Making a collage is a great tool for creating your context. Because your ideas are multidimensional, you will be able to visually create a representation of the thoughts and feelings that you are working with. This is so helpful for getting clear about identifying what you really want, especially as you fine-tune your context. It will also be helpful to express your feelings with your partner and birth team so that you are completely clear and aligned about all that you need and want for this birth. If you had difficulty in chapter 3 when you designed your context through words, you might find it easier to represent what you are feeling with images. For example, if one of the words you picked for your context is *peaceful*, pull images that relate to what you mean when you say "peaceful."

You can also create a collage that represents your vision of your lifestyle with your new baby, what your relationship will be with your child, or what your life will look like once the baby is born. The images can include how you feel about yourself, your career, your relationship with a significant other, friends, family, home, dreams, children, your creativity, and more.

To start, get a black or white poster board, some glue, and a stack of magazines or photos that you are connected to. Pull words and images from the magazines that match whatever you are creating, so that you can share with others exactly what you want your experience to feel and look like.

I do a collage every year—I call it a treasure map that includes every area of my life and what I am creating for the next year. It is also a great visual reminder to keep all that you are working toward alive in your mind.

Create an Energy Painting

My friend Kathryn Jaliman is an amazing artist. She created a beautiful painting for me that honors an experience I once had when I was pregnant with Savannah and meditating. She truly captured the divinity of that moment for me, and I use that painting to remember how it felt when I was pregnant with Savannah.

When Kathryn was in the early stage of pregnancy, she told me that she kept seeing a curly blond–haired, smiling child in her mind. She created a representation of that child's energy. To create your own energy artwork, put aside all preconceived notions about how good or how bad of an artist you are. If this exercise resonates with you, you are good enough! Pick up that brush, marker, or pencil or those collage materials, and let your spirit soar. Allow your child to inspire your strokes, your collage choices, your colors and forms. Work on this until you sense inwardly that it's finished.

When the picture is finished, speak to it, creating a connection with your child. Envision the child, and be "one" with him or her. Imagine that the child's vibration can be expressed in a certain color, form, design, or image and, without judgment, put that on the paper or the canvas. I recommend creating this artwork while you listen to music and, again, choose a CD that represents the energy of this child-to-be.

Another great project is to document your pregnancy photographically, creating a visual representation of how your body changes daily, weekly, or monthly. This is a wonderful present to give yourself and your children to commemorate this time in your life.

Movement and Exercise

A woman's body should be in peak physical shape for the birthing process. Unfortunately, many women view pregnancy as an exercise "time out." Although vigorous aerobic or strength training might not be the wisest approach, there are many types and levels of physical activity that are highly recommended for pregnant women.

Physical exercise during pregnancy has many positive results. First, it will keep your body open and comfortable, accommodating your growth as well as your baby's. Exercise increases the production of endorphins, which creates a feeling of euphoria and relaxation. It can also ease nausea, sleepiness, and other discomforts. Finally, when you experience muscular aches and twinges from exercise, you can practice pain-management techniques and see how they will work during childbirth.

"Shake Your Mood" Exercise

Any time you need to get out of a funk, increase your energy, or lighten your spirit, get moving. Breathe deeply while you get active. If you really want to make a shift from where you are to somewhere else, you need to purposefully integrate your thoughts, attitude, and actions so that you are brought into your most powerful state, the present moment.

Start by standing up and raising your arms as high as you can. Then quickly bring them down to your sides. Repeat for a minimum of ninety seconds, inhaling as you raise your arms up for a count of four, then exhaling as you bring your arms down for a count of four. Take deep breaths as much as possible. As your arms go up, mentally or vocally repeat, "Every day in every way" and as your arms go down, repeat, "I feel better and better—Yes!" You can replace the words *better and better* with any others that suit the mood you are trying to create. For example, choose *calmer and calmer, stronger and stronger, more and more peaceful,* and so on.

Take a Gratitude Walk

If you need to shift from negative to positive, take a gratitude walk. Start by walking energetically and rhythmically. If you are in a state of fear or anxiety, know that you can transform your mind by taking action, consciously breathing more deeply, and using your mental will-power to focus on a single idea: gratitude. Energetic walking will help reinvigorate your mind and your body.

To do this exercise, find a space where you can walk for at least twenty minutes without being interrupted by traffic patterns. Place your attention on your breath for one minute, consciously making it deep, regular, and even. Next, repeat the words *Thank you* and in between each *Thank you*, mentally create a vision of what you are thankful for. Keep harnessing your breath and your attention. If you start to get grumpy, worried, or anxious, go back to your breathing and start again.

Prenatal Yoga

Yoga is an excellent form of exercise because it strengthens both the body and mind. The word *yoga* means "union," suggesting that yoga helps to foster the conscious connection between the two main components of your identity. Elena Brower of ViraYoga in New York City believes that the human body carries the most precise intelligence; your task is to listen to it and yoga is a great way to do just that.

Prenatal yoga is different from traditional yoga because the postures are adapted to accommodate the transformations of the pregnant body. It will help you focus your mind and become aware of how your body changes as you progress through your pregnancy. Yoga can also help by offering you a vantage point of acceptance and abundance. The mind-body union that is exercised in prenatal yoga allows you to transcend the self and strengthen the connection between you and your growing baby. Your prenatal yoga practice will awaken your confidence and trust in your body, as well as your capacity for birth and motherhood.

The skills that you gain from yoga will also be invaluable during childbirth. First, yoga reinforces the importance of breathing when you are working through difficult incidents. It also teaches you to observe stressful situations first, rather than react hastily to them. Finally, yoga teaches the importance of maintaining focus. You will learn that difficulties do not last forever. Most important, you just might be pleasantly surprised at how mentally and physically strong you really are.

Like most things in life, all prenatal yoga classes are not created equal. Make sure that you choose a class or at-home DVD that matches your childbirth context. Choose a practice that is well monitored, clean, and has good "buzz" among other pregnant women. During each class, your yoga teacher will guide you through a series of asanas (yoga poses) that will stretch and lengthen your body. They can also alleviate the aches and pains related to pregnancy. Some of the poses will help build endurance.

You may find that the poses I discuss in this section are challenging, but as you build stamina, they will become easier. The key is to know when to let go. Hold each of the poses just beyond the point where you feel simple relaxation, until you feel the stretch going a little deeper. Don't push yourself to injury, but walking the line of strong sensation is fine. Don't hold your breath and wait for the pose to end; instead focus on the movement of your breath and observe the sensations you are experiencing in your body.

Elena from ViraYoga helped me design the following prenatal yoga practice that you can try during your pregnancy.

Pelvic tilting poses. These poses will keep the spine and hips mobile and receptive, increasing circulation in the pelvis and legs. When done on all fours, they will keep your baby off your spine, creating more room in your abdominal cavity, and encouraging your baby to move into optimal birthing position.

One easy pelvic tilt asana is called the *Cat-Cow Stretch,* shown in the photos on the top of page 125. This pose increases spinal flexibility and abdominal strength, and can also help prevent or mitigate back pain. Start on all fours, with your wrists underneath your shoulders and your knees underneath your hips. Think of your spine as a straight line connecting your shoulders to your hips, and of your neck as a natural extension of your spine. On the inhale, curl your toes under, drop your belly, and gaze up toward the ceiling. Let the movement in your spine start from the tailbone, so that your neck is the last part of you to move into the stretch. On the exhale, release the tops of your feet to the floor, round your spine, and drop your head until you are gazing at your navel. Repeat for five to ten breaths. You can also try switching the breathing to inhale as you round your back and exhale as you arch it.

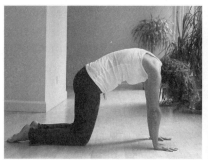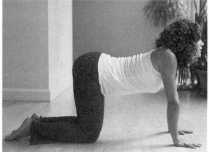

Standing poses. These asanas will strengthen the leg and seat muscles, which attach to the knees and pelvis. These joints are vulnerable during pregnancy because your body is surging with high levels of relaxin, a hormone that opens the pelvic and hip muscles in preparation for the birthing process. This hormone has a softening effect on your ligaments, creating the sensation of increased flexibility, which can lead to overstretching. Strengthening your leg muscles will help prevent injury and create endurance and confidence.

One of my favorite standing poses is the *Chair Pose,* shown in the photo at the bottom of the page. If you have yoga blocks, you will want to use two of them; place one between your feet to make sure they are parallel and the other between your upper thighs to strengthen your inner thighs and pelvic floor. Take a deep breath and, as you exhale, bend your knees and sit back like you are about to sit in a chair. Lengthen your tailbone slightly down toward the floor. You may keep your hands on your hips or bring your arms overhead with your palms facing each other.

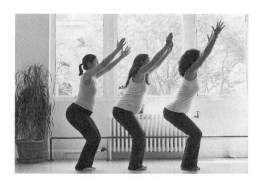

Another powerful standing asana is *Warrior II*, shown in the photo below. This pose will cultivate both mental and physical strength, as well as stamina. In addition, it will help open your hips to prepare for childbirth and lengthen your lower back, to keep your belly from shortening your lower back muscles. As you start to feel the sensation of the pose, remind yourself that you can overcome anything.

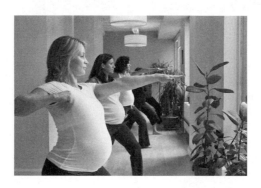

To do this pose, start with your feet hip distance apart. Step your left foot forward, planting it far enough away from your right foot so the distance encompassed by your feet is at least as long as one of your legs. Then, turn your right toes in and your left toes out. Take a deep breath and extend your arms, so that they are parallel to the floor. Your left arm should be straight in front of you, and your right arm will extend behind you as if you are shooting a bow and arrow. As you exhale, bend your left leg, directing your left knee toward your fourth toe. Lift your thigh muscles just above the knee to engage, and expand your chest from your collarbone all the way up to your fingertips. Breathe into your belly, with your baby's comfort in mind. Take a deep breath and as you exhale, straighten your left leg, keeping your arms out (or put your hands on your waist if you need a break). Then, turn your left toes in and your right toes out to rotate in the other direction. Again, lengthen your arms, inhale and bend your right knee toward that fourth toe. With your tailbone long, reach your right arm forward and extend your left arm back. Breathe. To finish the pose, take a deep breath and as you exhale, straighten your right leg. Turn your toes to face forward, put your hands on your hips, and gently walk your feet back to hip distance apart.

Triangle Pose, shown in the photo below, is great for strengthening the legs, back, and arms. It will also release tension in your upper back. Many moms-to-be enjoy the inner thigh stretch and the lengthening of the spine and back muscles. Begin this pose with your left knee bent over your left foot as in Warrior II, then straighten your left leg and point your right foot forward at a 90-degree angle. Bend from your waist, placing your left hand on your left shin or ankle, or on a yoga block. If you are more flexible, you can place your hand on the floor in front of your left foot. Reach your right arm straight up, so it is perpendicular to the floor. Gaze up at the right hand or down at the floor. As you inhale, extend the sides of your waist, especially the side facing the floor. As you breathe out, imagine yourself expanding in all four directions, through all four limbs. Come out of the pose, and repeat on the other side.

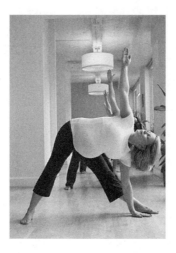

Abdominal toning poses. Many women think that the abdominal region is off limits for prenatal exercise. Not true! In fact, during pregnancy, it is even more important to maintain strength and stability in the abdominal core to help support the exaggerated curves of the spine and the weight of the growing baby. Carefully strengthening the transverse abdominal muscles will help you to push during labor and to prevent diastasis. The following poses are done seated or on all fours, not on the back.

Try the *Head-to-Knee Pose*, which begins as you sit on the floor with your legs extended straight in front of you. Bend your left knee and bring the sole of your left foot to your inner left groin, opening the left knee out to the side. Sit up on a blanket or a block if you need to, and press the back of the right thigh down into the floor. Lift your heart as you inhale, and as you exhale, gently fold down between your legs, maintaining the length of your sides and the feeling of openness in your upper back. On each inhale, extend the spine longer and on each exhale, deepen the forward bend but don't go so deep that your breathing cannot remain spacious and even. Repeat the pose on the other side.

Hip openers. These poses help open the pelvis to prepare for the baby's descent through the birth canal. They increase flexibility in the muscles that connect to the pelvis and can also alleviate common discomforts such as sciatica. Focus on some internal hip opening poses since the pregnant body naturally opens the hips externally, which contributes to the pregnant "waddle."

Try the *Wide Leg Goddess Squat with Arms*, which is a mini yoga flow vinyasa—a sequence of yoga poses done continuously, one after the next. Start with your legs in a wide stance, as you did with Warrior II. Inhale, while slightly straightening your legs and lifting your elbows. When you exhale, bend your legs and draw your elbows down three times. This is a good pose for opening hips, strengthening legs, and releasing tight upper back muscles.

Another powerful hip opener is the *Hero's Pose,* shown in the photo on next page. This is a seated pose that stretches your thighs and ankles and improves your posture. Start in a kneeling position. Keep your knees together as you separate your feet bringing your buttocks down onto a blanket, with a pillow or block placed between your feet. Your feet should stay pointed straight back, not inward or outward. Rest your hands on your belly, breathing into it. Focus on breathing into the back of your belly for ten breaths or longer.

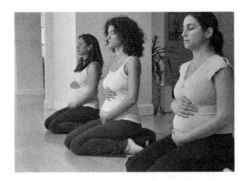

Gentle backbends/chest openers. These poses lengthen your lower back and strengthen the muscles that run the length of your spine. They also create a spacious feeling in your chest, around your heart.

Try a modified *Camel Pose*, shown in the photo below. Using blocks by your feet during the second trimester and blocks topped with a bolster during the third trimester. The basic pose begins in a sitting position on the floor. Come up on your knees. Draw your hands up the sides of the body as you start to open your chest. Extend your sides, from your waist to your armpits, in the stretch, then exhale, reaching your hands back one at a time to grasp the heels. Bring your hips forward so that they are over your knees. Let your head come back, opening your throat.

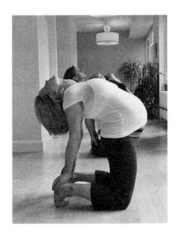

You can also try the *Bridge Pose*, if it feels safe and comfortable for you. Lie on your back. Bend your knees, bringing the soles of your feet parallel and close to your buttocks. Lift your heart up toward the ceiling and gently raise your hips, clasping your hands together and rooting them down into the floor or simply letting your arms lie on the floor, parallel to your body as shown in the photo below. Roll one shoulder under and then the other while you continue to lift and breathe into your heart and belly. To come out of the pose, release your hands and lower your spine back down vertebra by vertebra.

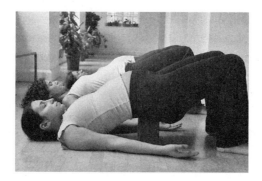

Supported Reclined Cobbler. The following pose can be done whenever you need to relax. You can also do it when you need a break during labor. For this pose, you may need two yoga blocks or small towels.

To get into this pose, sit in front of the blocks, facing away from them, with the soles of your feet together and your knees pointing out in either direction. Sitting tall, that is, with your spine straight, press the outer edges of your feet together. Then lean backward, bringing your elbows to the floor. Lower your back all the way down. Once you get into this pose, focus on freeing your breath and connecting with your baby. Stay here for a minimum of five minutes to feel the benefits of the restorative posture. With each breath, direct your energy inward and connect to the sensations of your baby and to the subtle energy working within you. To come out of the pose, roll over to your side and sit up, using your hands to support you. If you are not comfortable reclining on the floor, you may use the folded towels to support the spine. You may also want to place a block or a towel under each knee for support.

Kegels. A Kegel is not a yoga asana, but the name of a pelvic floor exercise. I call it an "invisible exercise," because you can do it without revealing it to anyone else. Kegels can help tighten up the pubococcygeal (PC) muscles, which can become stretched during both pregnancy and labor. These are the same muscles you use to stop urination. To do these exercises, tighten your PC muscles and hold for a count of eight, then slowly release and repeat eight times. You can do them anywhere several times a day.

Mock contraction. This pose, also not a true yoga asana, simulates the time of a contraction and can help you learn techniques to manage labor pain. To do this exercise, stand with your back against a wall and walk your feet out as far as the length of your upper thigh. Squeeze a block between your thighs and sit down like you are sitting into a chair. Hold this pose for fifteen, then thirty, then sixty seconds. Breathe as calmly as possible and smile, observing how you can respond rather than react, maintain your composure instead of backing out—great preparation for the birthing process!

If you are already familiar with yoga and maintain a daily or weekly practice, *the following asanas should be avoided during your pregnancy*:

Belly lying poses put too much pressure on the growing uterus and can cause distress to your baby. Avoid them following the first trimester.

Back lying poses or right side lying poses should not be done after the second trimester. The uterus can put pressure on the vena cava, the vein that returns blood flow from the legs to the heart. Blocking this vein can cause dizziness and nausea, and if you lie on your back or right side for more than fifteen minutes at a time, it can slow blood flow to the baby.

Deep backbends can place too much strain on the already stretched abdominal muscles during pregnancy. This can result in diastasis, a weakening and possible separation of the abdominal recti muscles. In some rare instances, the placenta can separate from the uterus prematurely. Deep backbends done improperly can also aggravate your lower back, if it is already compressed. Avoid doing backbends throughout your pregnancy.

Deep twists can be very dangerous, even from early on in your pregnancy, as they may compress your uterus.

Vigorous vinyasa sequences. These sequences can be awkward for pregnant bodies to perform and may be dangerous, as fast-paced movement can create too much heat in your body.

Balancing asanas pose a risk of falling and may encourage an improper use of abdominal muscles. They should be avoided from the moment you conceive.

Advanced inversions can create a risk of falling. Due to the relaxin hormone, which softens the tendons, ligaments, and muscles, the neck may be more susceptible to strain during pregnancy. Also, in rare cases, these poses can lead to an air embolism, which is a blockage of a blood vessel caused by an air bubble. The air passes beneath the fetal membrane and into the circulation of the subplacental sinuses. An embolism can be fatal to the baby or the mother.

Using Sound to Relax

In labor you may want to make sounds, and you should not care whether anyone is watching or listening. You need to feel totally uninhibited, free, and safe. I know that during my labor, at certain points it felt great to make noises, some of which sounded as if I were pushing heavy weights, while others were just sighs or moving through sensations or pain with my voice, riding it vocally. You can vocalize your feelings however it feels right, but one sound that resonates with many people is *Om*, the yogic chant. For many, *Om* is the birth sound. To make this sound, release your jaw, which echoes that movement in the pelvic floor and encourages the pelvic floor to release. This is especially important during labor when you experience contractions.

Om is not a word but rather an intonation. It is made up of three Sanskrit letters: *aa*, *au*, and *ma*, which, when combined together, make the sound "Aum" or "Om." It is believed to be the basic sound of the world and to contain all other sounds. It is a mantra in itself. To make this sound, focus on your breathing, and when you are ready to chant, take a deep breath in. On the exhalation, say "Om." Continue to make the sound through your entire exhalation, stretching it out.

Listening to music is equally relaxing. Notice how your favorite music supports all that you are creating. It can be a positive trigger to help you relax. When I was pregnant with my second child, Orion, the house was always busy, so I created a biweekly practice of having a prenatal massage to help me relax. At each massage, I wanted to listen to the same music. This practice always triggered me to relax and quickly go inward. I was so inspired by this music that I used it at various times during my labor.

Your musical preferences are as individual as you are. With an MP3 player, you can create your own toolbox soundtrack that features the types of music that make you the most relaxed or even energized. Be prepared with many different types of music: you never know what you will want to listen to during your pregnancy and for the actual birth.

Hands-On Relaxation

Touch should be reassuring and relaxing. During pregnancy and childbirth, touch can be profoundly soothing and informative. It is the most basic form of communication we have. With touch, there are no language barriers. Ina May Gaskin said that we are all born with "original touch," the state at which your awareness of touch is at its sharpest.

A baby born without the gift of sight will never lose his original touch because he can't afford to pull his attention out of his skin and his hands.

I created the following hands-on touch exercise with Raja Shaheen, the Reiki master who initiated me into the Reiki practice. The first thing most people do when they feel pain is try to get away from it. This exercise can help you deeply recognize where you feel sensations and bring a soothing breath to those areas in your body with the power of touch. You will learn to make breath a movement that can help you resolve pain. At the same time, you are learning to feel who you are in your body. Remembering the mind-body connection, recognize that your body holds all of your feelings and information.

You can do this exercise either sitting up straight or lying down. Place one hand on your belly, with the other hand above it. Breathe into this space and see what you feel emotionally and physically. Feel that you are supported, safe, and comforted. This part of your body represents your most visceral-emotional site, where you can recognize your essence, your vulnerabilities, your needs, your sense of self, your self-esteem, and how you feel about yourself.

Next, move your hands below your belly to either side of your pelvic bone. If you are sitting in a chair, your hands would rest in the crease of your thighs and your fingertips would be touching the tip of your pubic hair. Breathe into this space, and see what you feel emotionally and physically. This is a vital place—the place of delivery, the last "zone" for birth. If there are remaining fears in your mind, they may live in this area. Use this time as an opportunity to translate fear into a sense of wonder and appreciation.

Now, move your hands as you continue breathing into your heart. Bring your hands to your heart, placing one on top of the other. The heart is the center of your entire self, connected to feelings of love, grief, and nurturing. Take at least two to five minutes and breathe into your heart. See what you feel in this place.

Move your hands to the back of your head, and position one below the other, cupping the base of your head. This represents the limbic, most primitive part of the brain, which is all about instincts and basic survival. As you continue to breathe into your hands at the base of your head, recognize what this feels like for you.

Bring your hands to the top of your head. Continue the rhythm and awareness of your breathing, and recognize how your touch feels on the top of your head and what this brings up for you. This area is where you connect with the part of life that is greater than yourself: the universe, God, or whatever the concept of the Ultimate Reality is for you. You can visualize and sense positive thoughts and vibrations coming in through your head. Make this area a color if you wish; I like to think of white or gold or a mixture of both.

Now that you have recognized each part of your body, think for a moment of any intentions or affirmations you have been working on for this birth. Place your hands on top of your head, move them to the back of your head, and then to your heart, to your abdomen, to your lower abdomen, and finally "hug" your baby.

You can also do this exercise by allowing someone close to you to provide their touch.

Reflexology

Reflexology is a technique that will allow you or your partner to release tension any time during this pregnancy and even while you are in labor. You can use reflexology to relax yourself during the first five minutes of a meditation or whenever you need to take a break and decompress during the day. Conditions such as back pain, morning sickness, fluid retention, and constipation can be alleviated by reflexology. Reflexology can also help you make progress while in labor. A certified reflexologist will know exactly how to use this tool to control and regulate your contractions.

My friend Angie Clarke is a nationally certified reflexologist who often works with mothers during labor. She has provided the following lessons, which anyone can use. During this practice, you will touch pressure points in your hands and feet that directly correspond to other parts of your body. These areas contain thousands of nerve pathways that go through almost every cell in the body. By massaging specific points on the hands and the feet, you increase circulation and bring more blood to that area, which has a healing effect. This helps your body get rid of blockages, toxins, or deposits, creating better internal balance.

When you resolve circulation problems, you are actually cleansing and loosening up your entire body. For example, the base of your fingers (the bottom third of the finger where it meets the hand) relates to your neck and shoulders. Use your thumb from your other hand to rub this area, and see whether you release any tension in your neck and shoulders. Hold and press the area, and you can almost feel the tension release. Continue to knead that spot until you feel peaceful, allowing the tension to take its course and dissipate.

Whenever you practice reflexology, make sure your hands are warm and your movements gentle, slow, and smooth. Be sensitive to your touch, starting with a light touch. Be aware of your posture and the position of your body; do not cause strain. You can practice reflexology with oils. I found that many pregnant women have a heightened sense of smell and might find scented oils too powerful. Angie recommends using olive oil if that is the case.

A foot massage can make you feel grounded when you are in labor. Many pregnant women get swollen feet and ankles, and reflexology will stimulate the body to get rid of excess water that it has retained. What's more, the sensation is very relaxing, which will help release endorphins and allow you to have more consistent contractions. The tops of the feet between the toes and your ankles are highly sensitive to touch, as are the soles. The following directions were written to guide someone else who works on your feet:

1. Hold her foot with both hands so that your thumbs are on the sole and your fingers on either side of the ankle. Slowly slide your fingers around her ankles in a circular motion. Move your hands at the same speed.

2. Keep your hands in the same position, this time pressing in with your thumbs, letting them slide toward and past each other. Then, pull your thumbs back toward the edges of her foot, as your fingers follow on the top side of her foot. Work the entire sole of her foot in this manner. This can be repeated on the mid and lower foot.

3. Rub the top of her foot, using light pressure from the middle of the foot up toward the toes. Be guided by the spaces between the bones. Your fingers should slide up in a brushlike stroke. Slide them from the base of her toe to the tip, doing this three times on each toe. Cover all of the sides.

4. Gently move your fingers in the spaces between the bones, from the base of the toes toward the ankle. This area is also the reflex point for the breast. This same technique can be used to unclog milk glands during breast-feeding.

My Favorite Relaxation Remedies and Treatments

Think of the following list as a basket of goodies from which you can choose your favorites. These are all practices you can integrate into your weekly relaxation:

- Listen to relaxation tapes and music.
- Take a soothing bath.
- Create an ambiance with scented oils or candles.
- Create beauty in your home with candles, flowers, scents, and so on.
- Use the art of feng shui to evaluate your physical space according to the guidelines of the ancient Chinese masters.
- Watch empowering movies and DVDs of childbirth.
- Take dance classes, exercise classes in water, or prenatal yoga classes.

Relaxing Practices That Require a Practitioner

- Acupressure
- Acupuncture
- Chiropractic
- Prenatal massage
- Reflexology

Food for Thought

Karen Gurwitz, the author of *The Well-Rounded Pregnancy Cookbook*, is an expert in choosing and cooking the right foods for pregnancy. She believes that pregnancy is a great time to reexamine what you're currently eating and to start eating better. Choose foods that are the closest as possible to their original form. That means minimizing processed foods and trying to cook your own meals or eat freshly prepared foods as much as possible.

Many expectant mothers really do have cravings and food aversions, so don't be surprised if you look at some of your favorite foods in an entirely different light. Many women can't eat certain foods during pregnancy. Mainly, this is due to the women's heightened sense of smell. These feelings should be honored: don't force yourself to eat anything that is unappealing to you.

In terms of cravings, you can listen to what your body is telling you to eat, but don't go overboard. Don't let your cravings take over your diet—let yourself have a little bit of whatever you want. For example, if you crave ice cream, have a small serving. Feed your cravings with better choices. For example, craving ice cream may mean that you want something cold and smooth. If so, try a healthy fruit-and-yogurt smoothie with some added flax oil. This is a much healthier option that might satisfy your cravings.

Karen's one caveat is sugar. Many women crave sweets during pregnancy, and she suggests that you avoid these and don't fall into the trap of using replacement chemical sweeteners. Three reasonable options are substituting agave, stevia, or maple syrup for sugar. They can be used for baking or to sprinkle over oatmeal or fresh fruit. These alternative sweeteners will satisfy your cravings and won't affect your insulin levels as much as heaping on the sugar will. Also there are some very healthy products that can satisfy your sweet tooth. One that I love is a "super food," Xocai, a dark delicious chocolate that is very low in sugar, high in anti-oxidants and other health benefits, and low in calories. You can learn more about Xocai and purchase it at our site: www.BetterBirthbook.com.

If you experience nausea or morning sickness, eat only what you can keep down. Many women get nervous because they're eating only crackers all day long, and they worry that they are not getting the right nutrition. If crackers are the only thing that you can eat, however, then eat the crackers. Don't worry about getting your fruits and vegetables now. Just eat what you can. Your appetite will return, and you'll go back to eating healthy foods.

Karen also suggests that during pregnancy, you should feed yourself the best-quality foods you can afford. Choose high-quality oils, whole grains, fresh produce, and, whenever possible, local and organic products. Make sure that you eat a variety of nutrient-rich foods. Every meal should be full of color.

Seasonal fruits and vegetables support your organs on a timely basis. For instance, during the spring you might feel a sense of renewal and want to eat lighter. Fresh leafy greens that are full of folic acid and calcium will help you clear out your lungs and nasal passages and rid your liver of excess fat that built up during the winter. In the summer, berries come into season, so you have an opportunity to strengthen your immune system with red and purple foods, the blood builders.

You should eat lots of greens during the first trimester. This will ensure that you get the folates you need at this crucial stage of fetal development. As you move through the next few months, and especially in the last trimester, double up on recipes of freezable foods such as soups, stews, and chilis. Freeze half of everything you cook, in portion-sized servings.

Nuts such as pistachios, pecans, and cashews are excellent sources of fiber, protein, and healthy fats. Almonds are great for calcium and fiber; walnuts are particularly high in omega-3 essential fatty acids, which can help fight postpartum depression. Add omega-3-rich flax oil to smoothies or salads. For quick and easy salads, buy prewashed, prechopped leafy greens, grape tomatoes, and baby carrots. Create a snacking shelf in your fridge with these items, along with washed grapes, cheese sticks, and hardboiled eggs. Also, stock the freezer with prewashed, precut, prechopped vegetables, including leafy greens such as kale and broccoli, so that they are on hand and easy to cook.

The list of foods to avoid during pregnancy typically includes:

- Alcohol
- Caffeine
- Deli meats
- High-mercury fish
- Raw eggs (would include homemade mayonnaise, Hollandaise sauce, and so on)
- Raw fish or meat
- Smoked seafood
- Unpasteurized cheeses

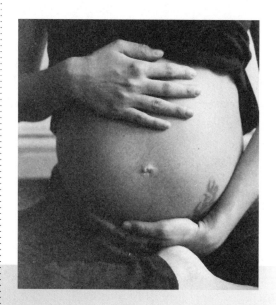

5　Connecting with Your Growing Baby

You have been working on creating and designing the context for your childbirth. Now I would like you to consider the context you want to create for your relationship with your child. Dr. David Chamberlain, the author of *The Mind of Your Newborn Baby*, has helped redefine the emotional nature of the baby in the womb. Dr. Chamberlain began his career as a psychologist who was fascinated by the effects of deep relaxation. He discovered that the human mind and the human memory were much more vast and complex than anything medical science was aware of up to that time. He has since dedicated his career to the field of prenatal psychology and the understanding of newborn memory. Over the last thirty years, he has been part of a group of pioneers around the world who have fundamentally redefined what we know about prenatal and infant emotional development.

He believes that beginning in the womb, babies are intelligent, conscious beings who are aware throughout the entire gestational period. This idea poses a whole new paradigm of infant and prenatal care. During the last hundred years, the primary theory of fetal development in our culture was based on brain matter. The prevailing wisdom was that the measure of a human being was the level of its brain activity. If, during pregnancy, fetuses didn't have their entire brains working, then they couldn't interpret everything that was happening. Therefore, they had no mental, social, or relational significance.

Psychiatrists such as Sigmund Freud supported this theory, calling it "infantile amnesia." Freud believed that humans don't really have significant memory capability until after their second birthdays. The medical community espoused this theory for decades. This way of thinking—in both the medical and the psychological fields—forced doctors and researchers to overlook the entire prenatal period in terms of emotional development. Obstetricians learned to ignore the senses and the mind of the baby because they didn't think there was any mind working. Within this paradigm parents were taught that the baby was little more than a passenger in the womb who wouldn't become "real" until a few years after birth.

We now know that this is not the case. Studies in prenatal psychology are now focusing on what infants can do, what their capacities are, and how early they begin to function. Current research findings point toward a completely different infant than obstetricians, psychologists, and parents were previously aware of. Today we know that the baby can think right from the start. Even in the womb, babies have a purpose. Their humanness doesn't begin after they are born.

If you look at pregnancy in this new light, your next logical conclusion is that the context you create for yourself and your childbirth is directly affecting your child right now. That is why it is so important to remember that whatever you do during the pregnancy contributes to this context. Every action needs to be consistent with your desires and wishes about your pregnancy and the subsequent birth. If you smoke, the baby smokes; if you drink, the baby drinks. Taking care of yourself is your first obligation to your baby and your responsibility as a parent. It encompasses eating well, taking prenatal vitamins, exercising, breathing, relaxing, and using all of the tools in the toolbox. All of these practices are designed specifically for you and your relationship with your developing child, and the time and energy you spend working at this deep level will pay off tenfold down the line.

As a new mother, you also have a responsibility to create a harmonious, relaxed, and healthy relationship with your child as soon as possible. I believe that parenting begins even before conception: all of the work you did to consciously conceive your child was part of parenting. The next phase continues throughout your pregnancy as you begin to create a bond with your child while she grows inside of you.

Connecting with your developing baby is one of the most important parts of becoming a parent. It initiates a bond that will last a lifetime. Yours is a unique intimate relationship: two people living as one. This bond is physical, emotional, and spiritual. By creating something deep and powerful, you will also affect the development of your child and make beautiful memories for both of you. This chapter will show you how to manifest this bond so that you learn to feel the life inside of you and begin to know this child.

The Mind-Body Connection and Pregnancy

During pregnancy, the mind-body connection is important in two distinct ways. First, there are chemicals that are released in your body that affect your ability—and desire—to bond with your baby. The most important is oxytocin. We will talk about oxytocin throughout the book, because this is the same calming agent that needs to be released for you to have a comfortable and relaxed childbirth. Breast-feeding also increases oxytocin levels in your body, which is why many women feel a powerful connection and a sense of relaxation while they are nursing. Oxytocin is even released during hugging, touching, and orgasm for both men and women. That's why it is called the happy hormone, or the love chemical.

In the brain, oxytocin plays an integral role in bonding and may be involved in the formation of loving relationships. Women naturally increase their oxytocin levels during pregnancy and throughout their child-rearing years. High levels of this chemical make women more relaxed and less competitive. Oxytocin also allows them to be more present to their families, putting all of their attention outside of themselves. Bonding with your baby will increase your levels of oxytocin, so that you will become more relaxed during your entire pregnancy.

This is particularly important in terms of the second component of the mind-body connection. Your current emotional world is creating your child's first environmental experience. Your thoughts, actions, and feelings directly affect prenatal development, both physically and mentally. In other words, your context is controlling not only your life, but also the life and the development of your unborn child. The latest research on DNA proves that our thoughts can affect what DNA replicates. Dr. Joe Dispenza, DC, the author of *Evolve Your Brain: The Science of Changing Your Mind*, who is known for his comprehensive understanding of the mind-body connection, said that the mother's emotional state encourages the development of the baby's genetic code.

For example, if you are stressed and anxious all of the time, you are releasing stress hormones such as cortisone and adrenaline into your body. These chemicals turn on your innate "fight or flight" response. On an emotional level, you are passing the same chemicals on to your child through the shared blood flow. Therefore, if a mother is stressed, she is warning the baby to be prepared for the same environment that she is facing. It's almost as if she tells the baby, "It's a dangerous world out there, and you can't be too paranoid." The excess adrenaline and cortisone that the baby receives will trigger physical, emotional, and biological changes. The baby begins to modify her genetic structure based on her mother's emotions. A stressed-out mom may produce a baby with a smaller head circumference, a smaller frontal lobe, and a larger hind brain. This same baby may become a child who is prone to react, rather than think through problems.

The Mind-Body Fix

If your negative thoughts and fears are affecting not only your reality, but your new child's reality, then you need to learn how to change them. People who live filled with fear have the potential to shed those fears. And when they resolve their fears and change their mind-set, they don't think fearful thoughts and they don't act afraid. Others can sense their fearlessness, freedom, sense of ease, peacefulness, satisfaction, power, clarity, inspiration, and more. In addition, they cease passing those fears on to their children.

As you create your new context, you need to transfer these same new positive thoughts and energies to your child. Your baby's personality is malleable, and it will take shape gradually. Its current environment has a particular effect, and there are some aspects of your baby's character that are inborn. You don't have the power to mold everything about your baby, so you should come into this new relationship as a prepared parent who is full of awe and wonder about your baby. Consider what she is bringing to you, what her purpose is, and how you can serve her purpose. This is what good parenting is all about: learning how the baby can help you and how you can help the baby. This emotional intelligence is not taught in schools. Unfortunately, there are no tricks to learning these lessons. You have to figure them out for yourself.

The first path to this symbiotic relationship is through creating a prenatal bond, which can happen in many different ways. Each of the following tools can help you transfer your context through your thoughts and feelings to your baby. By taking the time to move into a state of presence and love, you will send a signal to your infant that this is a safe and loving world, so that she can prepare herself both physically and emotionally.

Everyone benefits from connecting with your new baby: the baby, the mother, the partner, and inevitably the world. The communication you share with your child fosters development; the bonding also provides you and the partner with the beginning of an emotional connection and the first steps in teaching and guiding your child. Choose whichever way you are most comfortable doing this. You should dive into this new relationship and have fun doing it. The goal is for you to step into your new context and begin to communicate it to your child. By doing so, you will start to feel closer to the baby, and the baby will feel you. The partner will also feel the baby, and the baby will feel the partner.

You may even sense that it's possible to begin contact with the baby because the baby is already trying to contact you. If you can put meaning into this experience, so can the baby. This interaction will enrich the entire pregnancy. You are sharing your thoughts, feelings, and love with the baby, letting the baby know what's happening. You are creating a wonderful anticipation of a very real soul, communicating on a soul level.

When you and the baby are connected and you practice bonding throughout the pregnancy, the deep level of communication will show up during the birth. For example, I spoke to both of my children during different stages of labor. At one point, my son was moving a little too fast, and I talked to him about slowing down a little bit and said that we would work together, taking our time. I really was able to work with him as if we were players on the same team. I had the same kind of talk with my daughter during her birth. When each of my kids was crowning, I was able to put my hands between my legs and cup the baby's head in my palm. My touch communicated love; it was the first loving, physical touch outside the womb. I was in awe. There really are no words to fully describe the moment I shared with each of them. Now, that is an imprinted memory. Today, I always touch the tops of their heads, and I believe that they know on a deep level why it is so important in our lives.

Talking with Your Baby

Your ongoing conversations with your baby do not have to be spoken aloud, although they can certainly be conducted that way. What's most important is that you feed them love and support. As you talk aloud to your baby, he or she will learn to recognize your voice. This is particularly helpful for spouses or partners who want to become more involved. Lullabies you sing during pregnancy can be recognized by your child after birth, and some mothers report that these songs have an unusual power to calm the children down. The yin and yang of conversations is talking and listening, so remember to listen as well, to "hear" what your baby is doing and "saying."

Conversations, songs, and introductions to people you want your baby to meet can also be delivered in the form of a thought from your mind to your baby's. Some people would consider this type of communication telepathic, which means that it's directly mind to mind, soul to soul, heart to heart. If you are uncomfortable with this idea, then think of it as an internal conversation you are having, to which your baby is listening.

For example, when I was in the last weeks of my second pregnancy, my two-year-old daughter, Savannah, got the chicken pox. I told my unborn child, telepathically, "You can't come until Sunday, when Savannah will no longer be contagious so that she can be around you. Any time after Sunday really works better for our family. Can you please do this for me?" My son, Orion, was born on Sunday.

Nonverbal communication is a way to demonstrate your thoughts and feelings as actions. You want to be conscious and responsible for all thoughts and feelings, both verbally and nonverbally. These communications not only relate to upholding the integrity of the context you designed for your birth, they also relate to the context you create for the relationship between you and your child and the context you want to form for yourself as a parent. Nonverbal communication is also demonstrated by how you act. Often, you act without realizing the importance of what you're doing. But the way you act is part of your context, which you are constantly presenting to your child.

Connecting through Touch

The first sense a baby develops is touch. You may sometimes underestimate the value of touch, but for a baby, this is his main way of contacting you during pregnancy. When you touch him by touching your belly, he will want to reach out and respond. It may take a few weeks or months for the baby to be big enough to return your contact, but you should know that he intends all the while to return your touch.

I remember that very early on in my pregnancies, as early as eight or nine weeks, I could feel both of my children kicking. Other people told me that it was impossible, but I knew that I felt it. I later learned that when you touch a baby's head, all of your spirit comes through. Your love comes through, and your vibes resonate.

When you communicate with your baby, keep in mind that babies can feel everything that you experience, including pain. When they feel emotional pain, they begin to work around it, developing some sort of coping strategy. Babies can feel physical pain as well. For example, if a pregnant mother falls down the stairs, the baby inside of her falls down the stairs. If gunshots are fired at the mother, but she's not really injured, her baby can die as a result of the shock.

When surprising or unwanted events really upset you or your partner, your baby will experience them as well. You can help resolve the situation by continuing to have a positive conversation with him to explain the circumstances. In this way, you will create a clear relationship early on. You are letting your baby know that whatever happens in life, it can be handled within the parent-child relationship.

Meet Cinzia

When my sister, Cinzia, was pregnant with her second daughter, Charlotte (Charlie, for short), she often thought of ways to talk with Charlie and "touch" her. As a schoolteacher, Cinzia understood the importance of connecting with her children early on. She often touched the top of her stomach and talked with Charlie in her mind, and when she did this, she always found that Charlie moved vigorously.

Cinzia constantly read to her two-year-old, Alexandria, during her second pregnancy. Charlie frequently became very active during these daily "story-reading sessions." Cinzia felt that this was Charlie's way of communicating that she could hear the stories. Charlie is now four years old and is fully able to read. As an infant, she climbed into all of the books and flipped through them: she truly has a love of reading and books that started in utero!

Many other BornClear participants have told me about their own moments of connecting with their babies in utero. One woman said that every time loud music played, her baby began kicking in such a way that the mother knew the music was not appreciated. This mom could really feel the baby's upset emotions. Another mom told me that her baby was very active at 9:00 p.m. and again at 3:00 a.m. every night. The mom tried to connect with the baby during these times; now, the baby is two months old and still wakes up at those exact times.

One of my favorite anecdotes comes from a 1989 edition of *Omni* magazine. The story recounts a mother who loved the television show *M*A*S*H* and watched it religiously during her pregnancy. After the birth, she noticed that whenever her newborn son heard the familiar theme song, he stopped whatever he was doing and stared at the television.

Start Connecting with Your Baby By Doing What You Love

The diversions that you already enjoy can be used to connect to your baby. For example, listening to music, going for a walk, or creating quiet moments are all opportunities to bond with your baby. By sharing what you love to do, your baby will come to understand you. Also, when you work with the BornClear toolbox, you may discover new practices that become special during this time with your baby.

Creating Memories

Dr. David Chamberlain and others have recorded the birth experiences of many people. The following account is one of many that shows that the birthing experience and the relationship with your parents can still live in your life and your body. Some of these experiences can be called "birth traumas." I'm including this story so that you will consider the impact of everything you do and say and how you behave during your pregnancy. More than at any other time in your life, during pregnancy you are never alone.

When I was writing this book, I was introduced to a marvelous woman, Barbara Powers, who runs Amayal, a homeopathic health and childbirth education center in Monterrey, Mexico. She shared her birth experience with me. It was this experience that led her to create a unique center, located in the city with the highest C-section rate in the world: 92 percent. Mothers begin her five-month course when they are three months pregnant. Some of them come in even when they are only thinking about getting pregnant.

In curing herself of leukemia, Barbara Powers had to change her cellular structure and begin her life again with a completely clear context. With the help of an incredible psychotherapist, Armando Morones, PhD, she was able to return to her birth experience. She found that she had a lot of anger in her body. He took her back to see where in her body the anger resided and, in a general sense, to discover how far back a person can go to find out when he or she first sensed anger. It turned out that for Barbara Powers, the anger was present as early as birth.

Barbara shared her experience with me. "I started to see for myself that there was fear in the womb and that my father was expecting a boy and I was fourth generation, the eldest of the eldest, and they had all been males. So I could sense the fear. I was also able to sense the inability of my mother to feel anything, communicate freely. I could feel that she was not contacting me, and I was not in contact with her. Then I went through the whole birth process and felt why I did not want to come out. I was a forceps delivery, which occurred in 1940 when there weren't as many other types of technology as now. I could sense that I did not want to come out because my father was there in the room. I didn't want to come out because I knew that he'd be disappointed."

Barbara's prenatal experience shows just how early human beings can be affected by emotional imprint and how subtle and complex an unborn child's consciousness is. For more theoretical background on what is behind Armando Morone's work and Barbara's primal experience, check out Arthur Janov's books *Imprints, The Biology of Love,* and *The Feeling Child.*

Working on Your Relationship with Your Partner

One important part of your context is your relationship with your spouse or partner. Your unborn child can pick up the outward atmosphere of your relationship. She is literally conceived into that energy with a mechanism to cope with it, but she also has the ability to change her impression.

In psychotherapy, people are always going back to the origins of where they got off track in how they view themselves and their parents and even how they view life. We now know that babies can get off track right in the womb, as soon as a pregnancy is discovered. For example, if a mother finds out she is pregnant and screams, "Oh, my God, this can't be true. This mustn't be true. My husband will kill me!" the baby is already dealing with that reaction. Right then, some babies decide that they are no good, they are a hazard to their mothers, or they've got to constantly please their mothers because their very survival depends on it.

This doesn't mean that the experience is cast in stone, but it is recorded and it has to be modified. It doesn't just go away. Remember that the conversations you have with your partner, as well as the feelings that you carry within you about him, will be felt by your baby. Now is a great time to begin to resolve hurt and anger that are still present in your relationship. You should create ways to work through all of your communications with your partner, resolving issues and creating alignment on a daily basis. This alone is a conscious, amazing practice. Use the honesty log in the toolbox and the alignment process in chapter 8 to support your efforts in doing this. Call on any other resource you need to feel free and happy.

Naming Your Baby

When you bond with your baby emotionally, physically, and spiritually (whatever that may mean for you), you might be given signs in your dreams, experience visual sensations when you use some of the BornClear tools, or find yourself resonating with sounds you have heard. Being in touch with these signals may lead you to think of various names for your baby. Matching a name with this new little person, this life, this personality, this destiny, is a special process. Trust yourself and the journey.

Many of my BornClear clients have told me about certain signs that foretold what their babies' names should be. Some couples reported that their babies named themselves: that the parents were shown in various ways what the babies wanted to be called. Other people have meaningful family names they want to pass on, and some want to create a unique name that resonates for them. For example, one of my clients became obsessed with the story of Saint Anthony, the patron saint of lost souls. She believes that the presence of a child can bring your life into perspective, polishing off the wild edges, and she was looking to bring back her own lost soul. The father, however, wanted to have his child named after a flower and was particularly drawn to the chrysanthemum. For him, it is one of the most amazing and mysterious flowers, which looks as if it's hiding a special healing serum or answer inside its tightly held bulb of silky needles. Together, the parents were able to combine the power of a fearless saint with the magical mystery of a wild flower, and they came up with the name Cris-Anthony.

The stronger your connection with your baby, the clearer the answer will be about what to name him or her. See whether you can begin to recognize your baby's talents, abilities, strengths, and weaknesses without judgment. For example, my friend Patricia Schermerhorn works with women and couples on naming their babies. Her process is deep and pure of heart. Patricia said that most parents have no idea about the profound power and wisdom behind their babies' names. In her mind, children *are* their names: the name and the birth date convey the knowledge of a soul's experiences and the growth that was accomplished, coupled with the blueprint for a life.

Creating Pregnancy Rituals

You can create many rituals during pregnancy that are both fun and meaningful. Rituals have so much symbolic significance, are deeply memorable, and evoke so much emotion, especially when you design them yourself. Two rituals I love are making belly casts and throwing baby showers.

Belly casts are easy to make with the help of others. There are even kits available (see the Resources section at the end of the book). I made my own cast with gauze and plaster of Paris. You can have an event that focuses on making your belly cast—I made one for each of my children. When I was about eight months pregnant, I got together with some of my best girlfriends. We cut thick strips of gauze and wet them with plaster of Paris. We covered my skin with petroleum jelly first, then placed the gauze strips close together, from the base of my belly almost up to my neck. It was so much fun, talking and laughing while we created this memento of the pregnancy. I felt as if I was including the baby in the process as well. When it hardened, we gently pulled off the cast, which held the shape of my stomach and breasts. Later, I brought both casts to a foundry in New York City, where the owners/artists turned them into beautiful bronze sculptures that live in our home as artwork to someday be passed down to my children. This visual memory reminds me of how my children felt inside my belly, and it is a way for me to show them what we looked like and felt like. It is their first portrait.

Baby showers can be beautiful and meaningful gatherings to celebrate you, your family, and your baby. There are so many ways to create rituals beyond presents and desserts. At one of my baby showers, we created a ceremony in which all of my most-loved women friends gathered around me in a big circle—there were about thirty or forty women. Inside the large circle, four women in a smaller circle surrounded me, representing all of the elements—air, fire, earth, and water. One other woman led the ceremony. Through this ritual, we blessed this baby and our family. It was strong and so beautiful having all of that intention and love infusing and embracing us. Another ritual was that all of the guests at the baby shower held a bead for a bracelet we were making. Each person put a blessing on her bead for the baby and our family. All of these formed a beautiful bracelet that I wore while giving birth and still have now.

We then created a list of all of our family members and friends and built a "phone tree." Each person at the baby shower received the phone tree with a candle, and the instructions were that the first person on the tree was to call the next, and so forth, and so on, when my labor began, and each person would light her candle. Then the phone tree (the flow of calls in a specific order) would begin again as we announced the birth of the baby. This is such a great way to connect with all of your family members and friends, include them in the childbirth, and enable them to support you and communicate with you.

At another shower, I hired a belly dancer to teach everyone how to belly dance. The history of belly dancing is that it was the original birthing dance. It was playful and fun as I danced and held my baby in my big belly. We also served foods that were meaningful to me, and we played special music. All of this helped me connect and bond with my babies and celebrate them before they were born. Use these ideas, add to them, and invent your own. The most important thing is to take advantage of this time to celebrate your pregnancy and have fun.

Creating Community

Being around other pregnant moms may facilitate your ability to connect, feel, and communicate with your baby. Although it's not exactly a ritual, surrounding yourself with women who are pregnant can ease the anxiety you may be feeling. Use your prenatal exercise classes and/or childbirth classes to network with and meet other women like yourself. These classes provide a way for you to devote time to yourself, in an environment where you can connect with your baby. These communities should be supportive and loving.

It was always awe-inspiring for me to look beyond myself and see a group of beautiful pregnant women. I made it part of my weekly practices to attend at least two prenatal yoga classes a week—it did so much for me, promoting ease in my pregnancy and giving me time alone with my baby.

I know that my experience is not unique or anecdotal. One recent study by the University of California, Los Angeles, suggests that friendships between women are more than just special; they are healthy for you. Friends help shape your context: they add to the inner mix of who you are and who you are choosing to be. Scientists now suspect that spending time with friends can actually ease personal anxiety and counteract the stress you may experience, especially when you are pregnant.

This landmark UCLA study suggests that women respond to stress with a cascade of brain chemicals that causes us to seek out and make friendships with other women. This is an opposite reaction from the adrenaline surge described earlier in the chapter. Researchers suspect that women may have multiple ways of coping with stress beyond the "fight or flight" response. One of the study's authors, Dr. Laura Cousino Klein, proved that when the hormone oxytocin is released as part of a woman's stress response, it buffers the "fight or flight" urge and encourages her to tend to her children (if she has them) or gather with other women instead. When this happens, more oxytocin is released, which further counters stress and produces a calming effect.

This calming response does not occur in men the same way because of their testosterone. Men produce high levels of testosterone when they're under stress, which reduces the effects of oxytocin. Dr. Klein believes that a women's estrogen enhances the effects of oxytocin.

This study is important because it proves what many women have known all along: there is a reason why our friendships are so important. During pregnancy, it's even more crucial to connect with friends and encourage friendships, whether these are with women you've always known, such as mothers and grandmothers, or new pregnant women whom you meet. Your community of friends is part of your context. I like to call them "your tribe." In many cultures, there are tribes that form a community of support. Grandparents, village elders, midwives, and other women surround the new mother and her baby to support and guide them through this vulnerable and sacred time.

Create your tribe of women whom you can call on. It will include your friends and family members who can check in with you and who have experienced all of this before. They can provide support, love, and understanding. Having support so that you can take a mental, if not a physical, break with a friend can make you feel much more in control.

Moving On

Now you have experienced the first part of the BornClear program. You identified your fears and concerns and created a new context for this pregnancy. You decided exactly how you want this birth to take place. You have the tools you need to create a more peaceful and comfortable pregnancy. You have also established a permanent bond with your baby through sound, touch, and your emotional connection. Connecting with your baby in this profound way is an integration of your mind, body, and heart.

The next part of the program explains the more technical aspects of the birth itself. You will come to understand every aspect of the birthing process. Don't assume, however, that you can wait until the week before your due date to immerse yourself in this knowledge. You have plenty of work to do, so keep reading and continue to use the toolbox during the next few months of your pregnancy. Have fun with it! Enjoy this stage of your life, and take the time you need to fully understand all of the changes that will happen and all of the decisions that need to be made. Everything you have created and become aware of so far will help you "hear" and assimilate the rest of the chapters because you are becoming very clear about what you want and need.

PART TWO

BornClear
Birthing

Trust is the daughter of truth. She has an objective memory, neither embellishing nor denying the past. She is an ideal confidante—gracious, candid, and discreet. Trust talks to people who need to hear her; she listens to those who need to be heard; she sits quietly with those who are skeptical of words. Her presence is subtle, simple, and undeniable.

Trust rarely buys round-trip tickets because she is never sure how long she will be gone and when she will return. Trust is at home in the desert and the city, with dolphins and tigers, with outlaws, lovers and saints. When Trust bought her house, she tore out all the internal walls, strengthened the foundation, and rebuilt the door. Trust is not fragile, but she has no need to advertise her strength. She has a gambler's respect for the interplay between luck and skill; she is the mother of Love.

—*J. Ruth Gendler, author of*
The Book of Qualities

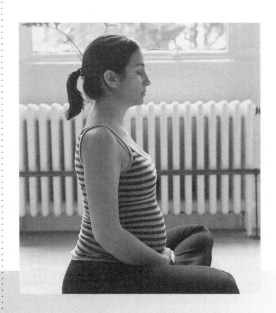

6

Accessing Your Internal Medicine

The first part of this book taught you how to choose your context for this birth and how to be mentally prepared for pregnancy. The rest of the journey focuses on your becoming mentally and physically prepared to live within the context you created as you prepare for childbirth. The first step is to completely educate yourself about the birthing process. My goal is to remove the mystery from birth to release you from the pervasive cultural and personal conversations new mothers are continually exposed to. These conversations are usually about the fear of pain. I find these conversations to be irresponsible and, worse, limiting. Birth will be a profound experience for you, and you need to focus on all of the various emotions and physical sensations that it will bring up.

I believe that if you have complete knowledge that encompasses the entirety of the process, you will be able to gain both clarity and power during the birth, so that you won't focus on the pain. The rest of this book will teach you how to work with your baby, your mind, and your body, to bring your child into this world, based on your context, in the most loving and comfortable ways possible.

It is important to read this material as early as possible in your pregnancy. This way you can begin to develop a general framework for understanding the birthing process, layered with your new expectations and ideals, while always keeping your context in mind. If you are completely comfortable with this information from the beginning of your pregnancy, not only will you fully understand your doctor's or midwife's philosophy and protocols, you will be in a better position to shape and influence your own.

Preparing yourself is exactly what it takes to powerfully deal with any new situation. Reading this material and understanding the process your body is meant to go through encompasses most of what you will need to have a satisfying birthing experience. You have done most of the necessary work to have the birth you want. Your knowledge of how the body works will inherently lead you to create the right conversations, align your intentions with your team, continue to live within your context, and, most of all, realize that you can trust yourself.

Understanding your mind-body connection and how you can effect and utilize it during birth is a very important element of embracing trust. You will find trust when you know you have done your best and feel that you are capable and ready. This chapter will explain how your thoughts can direct the release of chemicals within your body that affect you every day, and specifically during childbirth. The more you can understand, visualize, and even feel this amazing connection, the greater your mastery will be, not only for this birth but for the rest of your life.

Birthing Begins in the Brain

Before we review the physical stages of labor, let's talk about where birthing really begins. Your internal medicine chest contains the chemicals or the hormones that your body naturally produces, taking its directions from the brain. There are three important hormone groups for birthing: endorphins (the pleasure hormones), oxytocin (the love hormone), and prolactin (the mothering hormone). There are also hormones that can work against you, such as the catecholamines (stress or excitement hormones such as adrenaline, which includes epinephrine and norepinephrine). Each of these hormone groups is always present in the body, not only during labor. The trick to having a more comfortable birth is, first, understanding what triggers their release and, second, being able to control when they are released and in what quantities.

The powerful mind-body connection allows you to be in command of your internal medicine chest and to release more or less of each chemical as you need it. Your mental state can easily affect their availability and effectiveness during labor. By learning how to manage your thoughts, concerns, and fears, you can control these chemicals and use them to your advantage. You can then practice releasing these chemicals by doing the exercises in the toolbox. Doing so will make you familiar with mastering the mind-body state so that you can control what chemicals are released during childbirth. At that time, you will need to reach a point where you are "thinking less" (meaning less worrying or stressing) and "feeling more" (being completely connected with your mind and body).

During the beginning of the birthing process, the most active part of the body is the primitive part of the brain (the limbic area). This area releases the hormones that will allow your uterine muscles to respond: to open and help move the baby down and out. This intuitive part of the brain also controls your emotional responses. For example, the ability to stay calm and relaxed actually slows your brain waves into what is called an alpha state, in which it is virtually impossible to release adrenaline. In contrast, your awareness and thoughts originate in the neocortex, the most developed part of the brain. Your inhibitions grow within this area. Any stimulation of your neocortex during birth, such as exposure to bright lights, loud noises, emotional upsets, or even talking, will stimulate the release of adrenaline, which will inhibit the birthing process by shutting down the intuitive "birthing brain."

The goal, then, is to turn your environment—including your context—into a metaphorical space where you are safe and uninhibited so that you can continue to release endorphins in your body. Feeling safe may mean something different to each person, but it usually refers to the ability to relax completely, trust your choices, and be nurtured by your environment so that you can be fully uninhibited. Safe means that you are aware of gentleness around you and that you feel understood, respected, and even revered.

Let's look more closely at each of the chemicals in your internal medicine chest and see exactly how you can control them to create the birthing experience that most closely matches your context.

Endorphins. Whenever you are able to relax deeply, you release endorphins in the body. This can happen while you are working out, relaxing, having fun, having sex, meditating, or using any of the tools in the toolbox. During labor, the goal is to let go of your inhibitions and relax. When you do this, you are using your mind to work with your body. You are consciously harnessing your ability to release endorphins so that your labor can progress as it is intended to: in a controlled, fluid, and comfortable way.

Endorphins supply you with an awesome high during labor—a tranquil, condition. This euphoric feeling allows you to work with the intense sensations of labor and experience a natural distortion of time. Endorphins enable you to create a quiet, internally focused state of mind, in which you feel as if you are in a trance. For example, when you move through the first stage of labor (which you will read more about in chapter 7), your endorphins may help transform your state of mind from talkative, even social, and extremely alert, influenced by your verbal left brain, to a quieter, more introspective right-brain awareness. This shift from the left brain to the right brain facilitates the surrender that is required in active labor. Next, this hyper-focused state will distort your sense of time so that you feel as if you are completely in the moment and unconcerned with, and at times unaware of, how long the childbirth is taking. Mother Nature works perfectly to give you what you need at each moment of labor.

During my first delivery, I needed everyone to be very quiet; it felt like real time for them, but not for me. I was riding a wave and I felt inwardly focused, without a true sense of how much time was passing. I was in a beautiful, divine, quiet, knowing "space," where I could easily maintain my "surrendered" state. I was not helpless—I merely relinquished control and gave in to the labor process.

Endorphins are also natural pain inhibitors. In fact, medical science can supply no better pain reliever than your own endorphins: they are more powerful than morphine, and no epidural is more powerful than your endorphins. This chemical is thus very important during the stages of labor. During birthing, heightened adrenaline levels can cause contractions in the uterus even before the baby is ready to be born. At the same time, the stress response will stop the production of endorphins. So instead of letting you work through the pain and surrender to it by using your endorphins, your stressed-out body is literally moving toward a space of increased pain because it has cut off your access to this pain inhibitor.

If you have ever had a bad run or a painful exercise session, you'll know what I'm talking about. I find that when I'm running and not enjoying it, if I complain to myself, focusing on the discomfort and pain, I will tense up, as if I'm holding on to the pain. Sometimes the pain may even increase, making my complaining become louder. The more I focus on the pain, the more the pain increases and the more adrenaline is released. Yet when I allow myself to surrender to the sensation, and not hold on to it or focus on it, the discomfort will eventually morph into some other sensation that is more tolerable, or vanish entirely. This state of mind releases the endorphins, which will further help me deal with discomfort.

Oxytocin. Oxytocin is a specific type of endorphin, so it shares endorphins' opiatelike effects, inducing pleasure and a sense of well-being while acting as an effective pain reliever. I like to call it "the happy hormone." Oxytocin is made in the brain and is stored in, and released from, the pituitary gland. During labor, when endorphins surge through the body, oxytocin is also released, and contractions begin. Because sexual arousal releases oxytocin, some couples find that making love and/or nipple stimulation are two of the best ways to get labor started. If you can release large amounts of oxytocin during labor, it is possible to experience an orgasm during contractions or at the moment of birth. A wonderful documentary on birth called *Orgasmic Birth* by Debra Pascali-Bonaro showed some of these experiences, and many of the experts who were interviewed in the movie provided material for this book.

In any situation where you produce a great amount of oxytocin, whether during sex, birth, or breast-feeding, you must feel safe and secure in order to continue producing this hormone. When you become inhibited, the oxytocin production stops, and you may find it very difficult or even impossible to open up and give birth, continue to breast-feed, or have comfortable, enjoyable sex. This is another reason why it is imperative for you to learn how to relax and trust your body. By practicing with the toolbox techniques, you will again be able to get to the space where you are "thinking less and feeling more," which will allow the release of more oxytocin.

Catecholamines. If you lose or cannot harness a relaxed state, your levels of endorphins and oxytocin will fall. Your anxious emotions will signal your brain to release a form of adrenaline called catecholamines; these include cortisone, epinephrine, and norepinephrine. These stress hormones are secreted from the adrenal glands in response to stress, fear, anxiety, hunger, or cold. Their presence will cancel out endorphins, causing you to feel more pain. Catecholamines will also prevent the production of oxytocin, so that if you become stressed during labor, your contractions will stop or stall, prolonging the childbirth and making you more uncomfortable. For these reasons, you need to closely control the release of catecholamines during labor.

The "flight or fight" response is completely automatic—it is part of your innate physiology, which ensures your very survival. When this stress response arises during labor, your goal is to immediately produce endorphins and oxytocin. In short, you need to work on creating a relaxed state. By doing so, you will overwhelm the catecholamines with even more endorphins and oxytocin. The more endorphins you release, the more oxytocin is created, which will then kick-start the contractions.

It is entirely normal for labor to stop or stall. Your focus might be interrupted, or you might have an outside thought, or you could be concentrating on the pain. If you stall during labor, don't worry. You can use the relaxation techniques from the toolbox to help get yourself back on track. You can also stimulate your erogenous zones, such as your breasts or clitoris, which will automatically release oxytocin and reactivate contractions. This is yet another reason why it is so necessary to feel uninhibited during birth and to have privacy if and when you need it. The same light touch that produces goose bumps on your arms is all it takes to release endorphins. A light back massage or warm water also releases endorphins and oxytocin and can help jump-start labor again. Finally, see if you can identify what "interrupted" your labor in the first place. If it was a thought, try to work with that thought until you can stop resisting and surrender to the next phase of labor.

Moving into the Body

The baby is housed in the amniotic sac, surrounded by the placenta, which is enclosed in the uterus. The uterus contains both vertical and horizontal muscles that are directly controlled by the hormones mentioned in the last section. When endorphins kick in and oxytocin is released, the vertical muscles start to pull up, and, as they move, they nudge the baby down and out, supporting him as he descends.

The horizontal muscles are at the base of the uterus near the cervix, and they open like sliding doors. You can feel your cervix if you stick your finger up your vagina. It has a rubbery consistency and is about the size of the tip of your nose, although it can be bigger. In the middle of your cervix is a hole that will thin and open as the horizontal muscles contract—that's called dilating. Together, the movements by both sets of muscles cause contractions.

While the vertical muscles pull up, the horizontal muscles at the bottom pull back and open. They work together in a gorgeous design, in harmony. You can actually feel them moving if you focus your mind on your labor. You can visualize them as well. For example, at one point during Orion's birth, I felt him descending. Keeping relaxed, I focused my mind on the muscles, visualizing my horizontal muscles spreading at the bottom, my cervix dilating, and the vertical muscles pulling up and over at the top, gently nudging Orion down and out.

These uterine muscles need a continuous supply of oxytocin to do their work because if the catecholamines kick in, your muscles lock. If that happens, you will feel pain because the baby is stalled when he should be moving. More pain may increase your stress, which leads to more stalling. Another surge of oxytocin and endorphins is needed to break this cycle. This is another example of the human body's ingenious design: When the muscles lock the adrenaline has signaled the body that something is wrong. When you relax again, bringing your endorphin levels back up, the oxytocin will signal the contractions to resume.

The Power of Pain

There is no denying that you may feel some discomfort during the birthing process. Labor can be painful. But pain is your body's signal that something is happening inside; it is your internal navigator. Your sensations of pain will tell you when to push the baby. Or, the pain will alert you to refocus and relax so that you can concentrate on producing more endorphins and oxytocin. As mentioned earlier in this chapter, pain also raises levels of adrenaline and catecholamines, as a natural response to the stress the pain is causing your body.

Dr. Nancy Griffin wrote that the main cause of pain in a normal childbirth is often the fear-tension-pain syndrome that was described in the previous section. When your body releases catecholamines, the horizontal muscles in the uterus will contract. These muscles will stop labor by further tightening the cervix. At the same time, the vertical muscles will stop moving. The result is the very real pain of two powerful muscles pulling in opposite directions each time you have a contraction.

When you experience more pain than you feel you can handle, you have to bring your mind to the sensation and then focus on something else that is less painful and more manageable. The practice in the toolbox, specifically the physical exercises, the breathing techniques, and the visualizations, will teach you how to manage and work with pain. During childbirth, you will be able to call on whatever practices in the toolbox instantly helped you relax when you did them earlier. An effective practice could be anything that engages one of your senses, such as an exercise, music, a smell, or looking at a candle—a kind of meditation.

If you have done any form of yoga, you may have experienced this ability to work with pain. In yoga, you are asked to hold a specific pose that can become uncomfortable over time. Instead of focusing on the pain, you are taught to relax into the pain, melt into it, and over time it will either become another feeling or disappear entirely. It is a fascinating experience, sometimes quite intense and interesting to work with. In birth, if you are connected to the pain, you will have this same power of playing with it, to the point that you can understand and hear the signals your body and your baby are giving you. You will be able to follow your instincts and will know what to do while you are completely present to this truly amazing experience.

As you work with the pain of labor, your body will release oxytocin, and your mental environment will support your inward process and connection to your baby. You will become hyper-aware and will be able to clarify your priorities for dealing with the pain. I have since used this technique for dealing with other types of physical pain, including a recent injury to my foot.

The Role of Conventional Drugs

The powerful mind-body connection and the techniques outlined in the toolbox may be all that you need to progress through your childbirth. Or, your particular delivery might require the use of conventional medications or interventions. It is important to know what these medications do, even if you don't intend to use them. Many variables arise during delivery, so if you decide to use conventional drugs in the heat of the moment, you can feel secure that you are choosing from a knowledgeable and empowered state of mind. Whatever you choose will be perfect for you. There is no specific equation that I recommend, and I certainly don't believe that using conventional medications during delivery is a sign of a failed or less than perfect birth.

Most of my clients come to the BornClear class without understanding what these drugs truly are. For many people, drugs are the very thing that increases their fear, worry, or blame about the birthing process. But once people learn about the drugs' purpose and understand their pros and cons, including the possible side effects, they are able to relate the drugs more clearly into their context, instead of having a knee-jerk reaction when they are presented with options. At the same time, remember that with many of these medications, women already have the ability to produce the same drugs in a more natural form, right in their own bodies. This is why you need to actively practice the toolbox techniques, so that if you choose, you can forego the synthetic options.

It is important for medical care providers to examine the repercussions of advising women to use drugs. In the perfect birthing world that we are all working toward, doctors and nurses would pause and consider the effects upon the mother and the baby, as well as the overall impact on the birthing experience, when they suggest intervention with drugs or early membrane rupture simply because a labor is progressing slowly. Hopefully, as medical personnel become more aware of the mind-body connection, they will not continue to fall back on technology to hasten the birthing process and will use these tools only when it is medically necessary.

Pitocin

Pitocin is simply a synthetic form of oxytocin. In a hospital setting, if your labor is not progressing or if you stall once labor has started, you may be asked whether you would like to get some "help" to start your contractions again. That is what Pitocin is for. The positive side of taking Pitocin is that it will speed up your delivery. It increases the strength of your contractions and will help you move the baby down and out of the uterus.

There are, however, downsides to this medication. Pitocin may reduce blood flow to the baby and may result in the mother's bleeding after birth. More important, everyone generates different amounts of natural oxytocin, and your doctor won't be able to match the level that your body produces or won't be able to augment it. Because of this, the level of Pitocin that is administered is usually a very high dose. This fact alone causes many different outcomes. First, the brain senses the additional oxytocin from the Pitocin and will stop creating its own natural version, which slows down your natural rhythm of contractions and inhibits the natural sense of well-being and euphoria that comes from your body's production of oxytocin. Once you relinquish control of your natural medicine chest, you will not be able to harness the power of the mind-body connection. Pitocin is injected into the blood stream, not into the brain. The baby's brain also produces oxytocin.

And because the doctor probably can't match your natural rhythm, the Pitocin-induced contractions are stronger and more frequent than normal contractions. They might feel very painful or too forceful. This level of intensity beyond normal contractions may then require the use of other drugs to counteract the Pitocin, which becomes the catalyst for continued medical intervention. Some women report that the intensity of Pitocin is like "being hit by a truck." You can feel out of control at this point and, in some ways, the birth *has* been taken out of your control and is now in the control of the drug itself.

For example, my client Karen G. was given Pitocin during her first two hospital births. Her third child was delivered with a natural birth in a birthing center. In her opinion, the Pitocin that was given in the hospital caused contractions that were much more painful than she had during her natural childbirth. What's more, the pain caused by the Pitocin elevated her levels of stress, which then stalled her dilation.

Epidurals

The term *epidural* refers to the procedure in which medications are administered. Instead of taking them orally or through an IV that is connected to your arm, you are administered epidural drugs via a soft catheter inserted into the epidural space that surrounds the spine. During labor, local anesthetics, as well as mild doses of opiates, are often given. The drug dosages are determined by the mother's body weight and will seep from the mother's bloodstream into the baby's circulatory system. The point is to numb the lower half of the mother's body, from the ribs to the toes, to reduce pain. Many women report that the epidural allows them to be relaxed and calm and not in pain.

Having an epidural during delivery can completely change the course of your childbirth. First, once it is administered, the mother will be numbed from the waist down and must remain in bed for the duration of the delivery, which most people do not know in advance. Being mobile and working with various positions can be vital to having a good childbirth experience. During the delivery, a mother would not experience the strong final contractions that occur as the baby is birthing, meaning that the epidural may prevent a woman from recognizing the natural prompts that tell her what to do. And in certain circumstances, once you start with medical interventions, you may require other drugs. For example, epidural anesthetics can reduce muscle tone and prolong labor. Under the numbing effects, you will be less aware of your contractions and may not be able to efficiently work with them. Since labor is prolonged, it can then become necessary to administer even more Pitocin, leading to doses of pain relievers and so on.

By falling back on these medications, you are muting the signals your body sends you, and you will miss the opportunity to fully experience the birth of your child and all that comes with a natural childbirth experience. The epidural medications may inhibit the mother's production of oxytocin, which would slow down contractions and possibly stall labor. These medications can also affect endorphin levels, so the altered state of consciousness that women may achieve during natural childbirth would not be reached. Following the birth, the newborn must process these drugs through its liver, which is usually not fully developed at birth. In some instances, the drug metabolism will increase the likelihood of infant jaundice.

On average, 70 percent of women who receive epidurals during labor experience side effects, which can include postpartum urinary retention, severe backache, loss of motor power, prolonged first- and second-stage labor, malpositioning of the baby at the end of second-stage labor, hypotension, fever, shivering, nausea, vomiting, and itching. Very rare but possible risks include trauma to nerve fibers if the epidural needle enters a nerve; a drug overdose, resulting in profound hypertension with respiratory and cardiac arrest; and central nervous system toxicity, resulting from an injection directly into the epidural vein. Epidural medications can also cross into the baby's bloodstream and can result in babies having poorer motor skills and lower neurobehavioral scores immediately after birth. They can also cause a decrease in muscle tone and strength, affecting the baby's ability to suck, as well as greater fetal heart rate variability, which can increase the need for episiotomies and forceps, vacuum, and Cesarean deliveries.

Painkillers

At some hospitals, opiatelike painkillers are administered during labor. These synthetic medications simulate the effects of endorphins and include brand names such as Demerol, Nubain, Dilaudid, Stadol, Nisentil, and Sublimaze. They are administered either orally or through an IV.

As with Pitocin, using these drugs during labor will reduce the woman's ability to create her own hormones, and therefore may inhibit labor. These medications can also pass from the mother's bloodstream into the baby's system. Even though drugs initially ease the pain, when they wear off, the pain that is experienced will be greater and more difficult to manage than before—the analgesics and/or the anesthetics send a message to the brain that it no longer needs to produce endorphins. This is because when the drugs were first administered, natural endorphins were still present, slightly easing the pain.

If You Are Late

If your due date passes without any signs of labor starting, please don't worry. Instead, trust and be patient. There is no rush; childbirth happens in its own time. Due dates are not always accurate. If there is no distress to the baby, and both of you look physically healthy, trust the timing. Many of my clients were late. Sarah L., for example, was planning to give birth in a birthing center and was ten days late. She was healthy and the baby was fine, but the rules of the birthing center said that if she went past her due date by fourteen days, she would have to give birth in the hospital that was affiliated with the birthing center. As each day passed, she became more and more tense, which potentially stalled the labor even further. I asked Sarah to start using the toolbox more frequently each day, visualizing her baby being ready and her body opening. We picked a day that she and the baby would be ready. We chose Day 13, and on that day she was much more relaxed and began to dilate. By the end of Day 13, she went into labor and gave birth to a beautiful baby girl.

It's okay to just relax and let the baby come when she is ready. Most doctors and midwives will not be concerned about a delay in delivery until you have reached the two-week mark. At that point, they may bring up the option of inducing labor. Inducing is sometimes a choice and sometimes a necessity—you will have to decide what method best fits your context and the situation at hand.

If you want to try to induce naturally, do lots of walking and have sex. Semen contains the hormone prostaglandin, which can soften the cervix. Also, the body releases oxytocin during orgasm. Two orgasms in a row are known to bring the baby the quickest. Another way to release oxytocin is via nipple stimulation. You must, however, stimulate the nipples for long periods of time. The usual recommendation is fifteen minutes of continual stimulation on each nipple every hour for several hours. You can use a breast pump, as well as your hands. You can also try eating spicy foods or a lot of black licorice candy. Licorice contains the chemical glycyrrhizin, which stimulates the production of prostaglandins. In addition, eating lots of licorice might cause mild diarrhea, and intestinal contractions can produce sympathetic uterine contractions.

If you are stressed and tense, however, chances are that these suggestions will not produce the desired effect. Your body needs to be relaxed and calm for it to open. Maybe this is why so many women start labor in the middle of the night. Like Sarah, you can begin to visualize yourself opening, communicate with the baby, and practice lots of relaxation techniques from the toolbox. Take a warm bath, catch a funny movie (laughter releases endorphins), or stroll through the park. Anything that quiets the mind will be helpful.

Acupuncture can help as well. One study conducted by the Department of Obstetrics and Gynecology at the University of Vienna demonstrated that acupuncture increased cervical ripening at term. If you choose to engage the help of experts, allow them to be, first and foremost, a resource or a voice of support. Continue to do your own thinking, to trust yourself and your own journey. You are your own most reliable guide.

There are some risky situations that require induction by a caregiver to protect the safety of you and your baby. If any of the following should occur, alert your physician or midwife immediately:

- If the membrane has released and labor has not started
- If the mother has highly elevated blood pressure
- Fetal distress
- The presence of a significant amount of meconium in the amniotic fluid
- A deficiency in the functioning of the placenta
- Excessive vaginal bleeding
- Indication of an infection or a fever
- Evidence of a prolapsed cord

Your doctor or midwife may have other methods of inducing labor as well. One technique is called "stripping the membrane" (it's also called "sweeping" or "massaging the membrane"). This procedure must be performed by a midwife or a doctor, who will stick his or her finger into the cervical opening and rotate it 360 degrees. By doing this, the midwife is facilitating the release of prostaglandins from the membranes and from the cervix (the same hormones that are present in semen). This action helps the cervix to "ripen" and open. In most cases, this procedure is done during an office visit. You're then sent home to wait for labor to start, which still may take a few days. Some women reported that they experienced intense contractions after the membrane had been ruptured. Again, remember that this technique can force your body into a labor that it may not be ready for. Maintaining an intact membrane can ease the impact of your contractions, as well as allow for the baby's head to be cushioned as it makes its way down the birth canal.

Sometimes hospitals or doctors have automatic "schedule induction for labor" protocols, and they do not always tell their patients when they begin this procedure. Medications are sometimes given to begin the induction process. Synthetic prostaglandins can be administered vaginally in a hospital. (One of these synthetic prostaglandins, misoprostol or Cytotec, is sometimes used for induction in the United States, even though it has a number of very serious risks and has not been approved for this use by the FDA.) Or, instead of using medication to ripen your cervix, your practitioner may insert a Foley catheter into your cervix with a very small uninflated balloon at the end of it. When the balloon is inflated with water, it puts pressure on your cervix, stimulating the release of prostaglandins, which causes the cervix to open and soften. When your cervix begins to dilate, the balloon falls out and the catheter is removed.

If your cervix is at least a few centimeters dilated, your ob-gyn or midwife may rupture the membrane by inserting a small, plastic-hooked instrument through the cervix to break your amniotic sac. If your cervix is very ripe and ready for labor, there's a small chance that rupturing the membranes will be enough to get your contractions going. If that doesn't happen, you will be given Pitocin through an IV.

The decision to induce labor is not one that should be taken lightly. In fact, it is one of the most drastic ways of intervening in the natural process of pregnancy and childbirth. However, Dr. Mardsen Wagner points out that there are certain specific conditions when inducing labor has been proven to save lives—serious intrauterine growth retardation (the baby is too small for its gestational age), documented placental malfunction (the placenta is losing its ability to adequately nourish the fetus), and deteriorating preeclampsia (a serious condition associated with the mother's rising blood pressure). Macrosomia (the baby is too big) has also been used as a rationale for induction, but data do not support this argument. Instead, research shows that when labor is induced in these cases, more C-sections are performed, with no improvement in perinatal outcomes. The bottom line is, if someone is suggesting induction, make sure that you have all the facts so that you can make an informed decision.

Meet Mia

Induction can sometimes involve looking at everything that might be preventing labor from happening. You need to discover whether you trust yourself, feel relaxed, and feel safe, and whether you are able to surrender and know what you really need and want, in order to allow the process to begin at the perfect time. On occasion, it takes introspection that goes beyond the mere mechanics of asking these questions. For example, my client Mia was getting ready for her second birth, but it was her first home birth. She was about ten days past her due date, so she discussed a course of action with her midwife, Cara. They agreed that Cara would sweep her membranes, which they did in Cara's office the next day while a group prenatal visit was being held. The speaker was a well-known acupuncturist, who found herself ready and willing to perform a serendipitous labor induction.

But even with these two interventions, a few days went by and nothing had happened. The next step that Cara recommended was for Mia to take a single tablespoon of castor oil, with instructions to take a second dose about six hours later. Cara later spoke with Mia to find out how she was doing and learned that Mia had become distracted by friends who had come over, and had never taken the second dose.

Cara could sense that there was a psychological aspect to what was happening—or not happening. She tried to intuit what she thought Mia would need to let go, feel safe, and let herself begin to labor. Cara decided to go to Mia's house to check on her. When she arrived, Mia offered her a cup of tea. Cara could feel that Mia was trying to really connect with her. They talked about photos on the refrigerator and Mia's family and chatted and connected like friends. Cara knew this was what Mia needed.

That evening Mia went into labor—she ended up having an "orgasmic" birth: with each physiological push, she said, "This is not bad at all," and afterward revealed that with each push she had a flood of pleasure that diminished the pressure and the pain of the descending baby's head.

Your Internal Medicine Chest after the Birth

In his groundbreaking book *The Truth about Newborns*, Dr. David Chamberlain said, "Mothers know deep within themselves what scientists are just discovering—that relations between mother and babies are mutual, reciprocal, even magical." Mothers in all cultures have been known to hold their new babies to their left breasts immediately after birth. Many of my clients tell me that in this position, they feel that "dormant intelligences" are activated, and that they seem to be flooded with instinctive knowledge on what to do and how to communicate with their babies.

There may be scientific evidence that supports their claim, as well as proof of the need for contact between mother and child. Immediately after birth, oxytocin is released by both the mother and the baby, and you may feel an instinctive need to cuddle or hold your child. Dr. Michel Odent explained that oxytocin stimulates the release of a chemical messenger, an atrial natriuretic peptide. He believes that this chemical, released by the mother, helps the baby regulate her own body temperature, metabolic rate, hormone and enzyme levels, heart rate, and breathing. The senses of taste, smell, and hearing play an important role in her being able to identify her mother immediately after birth.

The high levels of oxytocin that are present will cause you to become familiar with the unique odor of your infant, and, once attracted to it, you will notice that you prefer your own baby's odor above all others. The baby is similarly imprinted, deriving feelings of calmness and pain reduction from the mother. This extraordinary sense of smell will help the baby find your nipple, which has a similar but slightly different odor than the amniotic fluid.

Frequent body contact and other nurturing acts by parents produce a constant elevated level of oxytocin in the infant, which in turn provides a valuable reduction in her stress-hormone responses. When an infant does not receive regular oxytocin-producing responsive care, the resultant stress responses cause elevated levels of the stress hormone cortisol. Many psychological studies have demonstrated that low levels of oxytocin at birth can control the permanent organization of the stress-handling portion of the baby's brain, forming personality characteristics that will continue into adolescence and adulthood. Such insecure characteristics include antisocial behavior, aggression, difficulty in forming lasting bonds, mental illness, and a poor ability to handle stress.

Fathers are also a part of the oxytocin equation. A father's oxytocin levels rise toward the end of his mate's pregnancy. When the father spends significant amounts of time in contact with his infant, oxytocin encourages him to become more involved in the ongoing care. High oxytocin in the father also increases his interest in physical contact with the mother. In this way, nature has provided a way for the father to become more engaged and devoted to the family.

The Importance of Breast-Feeding

You will continue to produce elevated levels of oxytocin as a consequence of nursing and holding your infant; the levels are based on the amount of contact between the two of you. This hormonal condition fosters a sense of calm and well-being. As you might expect, oxytocin levels are higher in mothers who exclusively breast-feed than in those who use supplementary bottles. While the baby will make her own oxytocin in response to nursing, you will also transfer yours to her in your milk.

Immediately following the birth, your baby will be ready to breast-feed, if you choose to do so. Breast-feeding offers a wonderful opportunity for you to bond with her. At the same time, you are providing her with everything she needs: proper nutrition, warmth, and love. The decision about whether you will breast-feed rests solely on you because you will be doing all of the work. Fathers and partners can be part of the decision making, and they can take on other tasks besides nursing (bathing, for example).

In the last stage of labor, you will give birth to the placenta (see chapter 7), and your brain will signal your body to release two important hormones: prolactin and oxytocin. Prolactin is the hormone that's necessary to create breast milk. When it is released, you'll find that you experience a wave of instant relaxation. Oxytocin is called in to release or "let down" the breast milk into the mammary glands.

Your breasts will not look much different immediately after the birth because it takes a few days for true breast milk to come in. In the meantime, a nursing baby will receive colostrum, a thick clear liquid that is high in antibodies, some of which she cannot get any other way. These antibodies protect her from illnesses she currently has or has been exposed to. It will also act as a laxative to clean the meconium out of her body. Again, this was all beautifully designed by nature.

Between the second and sixth day after birth, the colostrum will begin to thin as your milk comes in. Your milk contains the optimum balance of nutrients and antibodies to support your baby's growth and development. No better food for your baby can be manufactured than your breast milk (even another woman's breast milk is not an equal substitute). Today, more than 60 percent of newborns are breast-fed, and this number is increasing every year. The American Academy of Pediatrics now recommends breast milk over formula as the exclusive food for infants up to six months old and advises that breast-feeding continue for a minimum of twelve months. The content and the consistency of your breast milk also change as your baby grows and develops. Breast milk continues to provide her with exactly the right mixture of nutrients to fully support her growth and help her deal with environmental changes.

Some women worry about their babies not receiving enough nourishment. It is normal for the baby to lose a bit of weight before your breast milk comes in. With my son, Orion, it took a handful of days for my milk to come in, and he did lose some weight, but when my milk came in, he was such a good eater that within a week or two, he gained weight exponentially.

Once your milk comes in, you may notice that your breasts get larger and more tender. This is called engorgement, and although the tenderness is uncomfortable at first, it will go away. As you're nursing, you'll notice that the rest of your body is changing as well. Breast-feeding will help your body return to its pre-pregnancy shape because it releases hormones that contract the uterus and prevent excess bleeding. Breast-feeding naturally engages your body's current fat stores, so you will lose your pregnancy weight more quickly, especially if you nurse for more than four months. Most important, studies have shown that women who breast-feed have a lower risk of developing breast cancer and osteoporosis later in life.

Emotionally, you'll find that breast-feeding enhances the bond you create with your new baby because it guarantees lots of holding and touching. These are the sensations babies need to feel safe and secure in their new world. For you, breast-feeding can help balance your mood, especially if you are experiencing postpartum depression. The constant release of prolactin and oxytocin during nursing will allow you to slow down and relax, so that you can rest and recharge. I breast-fed each of my children for eighteen months. Neither has ever had an ear infection, and, overall, both have been amazingly healthy. Aside from how convenient it was, breast-feeding was a precious bonding experience.

As your baby gets older and continues to grow, the benefits of breast-feeding also continue. Studies have shown that breast-fed infants are less likely to become sick and will have fewer digestive or respiratory issues. Other studies have shown a link between breast-feeding and decreased rates of contracting infectious illnesses and diseases, including diarrhea, ear infections, allergies, bacterial meningitis, SIDS (sudden infant death syndrome), diabetes, obesity, asthma, and possibly some childhood cancers. Long-term studies have also shown that breast-feeding for up to a year may increase your child's IQ and protect her from certain chronic diseases, such as ulcerative colitis, Crohn's disease, Hodgkin's disease, and liver disease.

This book is not intended to be an instruction manual on breast-feeding, so I suggest that you pick up one that is. A terrific resource is the book *Mama Knows Breast* by Andi Silverman. She believes, as I do, that the key to success in breast-feeding is trying different methods until you find what works for you. Have a sense of humor about it, and don't give up.

As you learn about breast-feeding, remember that you need to give yourself time to master this skill. Breast-feeding is hard work for both you and your baby to figure out. Most important, always ask for help. Lactation consultants, the La Leche League, pediatricians, midwives, hospital nurses, postpartum doulas, baby nurses, and friends and family are all resources whom you can call on. These women are now part of your tribe. There are breast-feeding support groups and online communities that can offer advice and guidance. You can also take a breast-feeding class (such as those given by the La Leche League) while you are pregnant, or you can watch breast-feeding DVDs. These resources are listed at the end of the book.

Practical Pros of Breast-Feeding

- You can feed your baby anytime, anywhere.
- You don't have to prepare a bottle.
- You don't have to clean or sterilize bottles.
- You might not get your period for a while.
- Breast-feeding costs a lot less than formula does.
- Breast-feeding is good for the environment.

Not-So-Practical Cons of Breast-Feeding

- No one else can do your job.
- You may risk sleep deprivation.
- You may have to use a breast pump.
- You will have to get used to feeding in public.
- You can drink alcohol and caffeine only in moderation.
- You may experience leakage.
- Your husband or partner has to share your breasts with someone else.
- Your husband or partner may feel left out of the baby-bonding process.
- You may experience initial discomfort.

I've found that the following tips made breast-feeding more manageable from the start:

1. *Create a nursing station in your home where you most like to nurse.* Choose a comfortable, supportive chair near a table where you can place a glass of water, a snack, nursing pads, and a burp cloth.

2. *Find a breast-feeding mentor after the birth.* Find a woman you know who has breast-fed, and ask her to help you, especially for the first few days. Your midwife or doctor will have resources such as a lactation consultant or a postpartum doula (see chapter 8) who will also be available to you.

3. *Make sure to feed yourself while you feed your baby.* You'll need at least 300 more calories per day than during your last trimester to keep up your strength and your milk supply. If you are exercising, add another 100 to 150 calories. And don't forget to drink plenty of water: breast milk is more than 87 percent water, so drink up!

4. *Catch and correct problems early on.* You'll know when breast-feeding isn't going well because it will become very painful for you. Most of the time, the problem can be fixed by changing your position or the baby's. The sooner you address the issue, the happier everyone will be.

Understanding Postpartum Depression

Your mind-body connection supplies an ongoing flow of information and reactions that doesn't end when your new baby is born. As a new mother, you will continue to produce high levels of oxytocin, which helps you continue to bond with and protect your children throughout their lives.

For some women, the emotional roller coaster that follows delivery is more than they can handle. Studies show that up to 30 percent of all new mothers experience postpartum depression. This high rate has nothing to do with how you felt about being pregnant or giving birth. Postpartum depression is a very real condition that happens to many types of women, regardless of whether they were "happy" or "unhappy" before they gave birth.

No one knows exactly what causes postpartum depression. Some believe that your birth experience may contribute to it. Another factor may be your fluctuating hormone levels, which affect mood and energy. Your estrogen and progesterone levels increase during pregnancy, and they drop suddenly after delivery. In some cases, your thyroid hormone level may decrease as well. These rapid hormone shifts may affect the brain's chemistry in a way that can lead to sadness, a low mood, and depression. Stress hormones may have affected your mood as well. The postpartum period is one of the most stressful and demanding times in a woman's life. Fathers, partners, and adoptive parents can experience postpartum depression as well.

Brooke Shields is probably the most famous woman in recent times who was willing to talk about her postpartum depression. Her feelings of shame, secrecy, helplessness, and despair were classic signs of postpartum depression. She found that these emotions began about two or three weeks after the birth of her first child, Rowan.

Many doctors and researchers believe that one or more of the following risk factors may predispose you toward getting this illness. These risk factors do not cause postpartum depression; you might have a number of them and never get depressed. Or, you may not have any of these problems and might still fall into a state of depression. If you do experience these problems, however, you can take the necessary steps before you deliver your baby to ensure that you have the help you need if the situation arises.

- Previous postpartum depression
- A family history of anxiety or depression
- An unplanned pregnancy
- An unsupportive spouse
- A recent separation or divorce
- A major loss during the last two years
- Complications at birth
- Other environmental stressors

Luckily, the treatment for postpartum depression is often extremely effective. Treatment typically involves a combination of therapy and medication. You can also use some of the relaxation practices in the toolbox to help you feel better. Interestingly, Brooke Shields has reported that breast-feeding was one thing that helped her beat this depression. She said, "I attribute a lot [of my recovery] to breast-feeding, because, for me, the physical connection is what I really needed, whether I enjoyed it or not. Somewhere along the line it was undeniable that she was stuck to me. I think that was important to my recovery." Breast-feeding would have caused her body to release oxytocin and prolactin, as discussed in the previous section, and that may have also helped her overcome the depression.

While it is certainly too early to worry whether you will suffer from postpartum depression, the point is that for many women it is a normal response to the end of their pregnancy, and it may be affected by the mind-body connection. You will have been pregnant for nine months, growing a little person and then birthing him. Getting rest, good nutrition, and exercise; continuing your relaxation practices; and surrounding yourself with lots of support are all necessary in your life after the baby is born. Be patient and loving with yourself. Relaxation of any kind is beneficial. Use the toolbox if you need help during this time. Your understanding of the mind-body connection will allow you to balance yourself after childbirth, just as it will at any other point in your life. Understanding yourself, your mind, and your body will enable you to become balanced emotionally, physically, and spiritually. This balance will promote feelings of satisfaction, happiness, and peace.

Meet Julia

One of my clients, Julia, was obsessed with her pregnancy. She read about birth, talked about birth, attended every one of her prenatal visits, went to birth classes, and talked to her doctors endlessly about her desire for a natural birth. Yet despite all of her hard work in developing her context, her delivery did not go as she had envisioned. In the hospital, she felt that her desires were whisked away by the dismissive attitude of her doctor and birth team. She underwent constant fetal monitoring, an enema, an epidural, constant negative suggestions that were not supportive of all that she was creating or feeling, and multiple internal exams, until finally the baby was born. By the end of the delivery, she felt as if she were simply a vessel, a piece of medical machinery for the doctors to direct and adjust. Needless to say, Julia was very upset and felt devastated.

Julia hoped that life would improve after she had her baby. She convinced herself that now that she had her baby and everyone was healthy, she could put her birthing experience behind her. But when she changed from being a self-confident, outgoing, outspoken entrepreneur to a woman on the verge of agoraphobia, she had to stop and wonder. At first, she was surprised that her therapist diagnosed her with a mild form of post-traumatic stress disorder (PTSD). Then she put the pieces together for herself: she could no longer drive on highways, take elevators, take subways, or get stuck in traffic. Was it PTSD, or was she slowly losing her mind? In actuality, she was suffering from postpartum depression. There was no question in Julia's mind that her birthing experience, the upset and devastation contributed to her suffering.

During her second pregnancy, Julia noticed that she was short-tempered and annoyed at everything. With the assistance of an amazing birth team, she was able to emotionally carry on with her pregnancy. Her therapist, her acupuncturist, two new midwives, her husband, her sister, and her friends were all instrumental in keeping her psyche well-balanced during the dark months of her last trimester.

In complete contrast to her first birth, her second son was literally born in midair. Julia told me that he came so quickly, the midwife didn't have time to put on her gloves. This time Julia labored naturally: in a tub, a shower, and her husband's arms.

Only through her second childbirth experience was she able to heal the first one.

What Fathers or Partners Are Experiencing

Men have their own internal medicine chests. Although they also produce endorphins and oxytocin in many of the same circumstances that women do, they also produce a pituitary hormone called vasopressin, which is what allows men to become more present and begin to bond and feel love. Men who are the best parents have high amounts of vasopressin. Released in response to touch, vasopressin promotes bonding between the father and the mother, helps the father recognize and bond with his baby, and makes him want to be part of the family.

If the father is living in stress or fear, however, and is producing lots of adrenaline, he can't generate vasopressin. To make that chemical, the father needs to get clear on his motivation to provide for a child.

A second hormone, prolactin, is also released by the father (and by you) during sleep. You will release prolactin in response to suckling, which promotes milk production as well as maternal behavior. For fathers, prolactin fosters caregiving behavior. Your partner's prolactin levels began to elevate during your pregnancy, but they will increase on their own after he spends a few days living with the new baby.

Using Your Internal Medicine Chest as a Life Tool

A strong, healthy mind helps to build a strong, healthy body. Once you have arrived at a place of peace and have an easy understanding of how your mind and body work in tandem, you can use this knowledge every day of your life or in any situation as needed. Your mind-body connection can help you feel satisfied and calm, as well as help you heal yourself if you need to.

For example, visualization is more than merely a tool that will help you relax. My good friend Patricia was once hospitalized with a very rare bone condition in her arm. The night before she was scheduled to have surgery, Patricia asked her father, who was very skilled and disciplined in the mind-body connection, to work with her. Using a relaxing tone of voice, he helped her visualize an army of men working on repairing her arm. The visualization was so clear and focused on healing that the next morning there was a remarkable difference in the condition of her arm. Patricia's infection ultimately healed on its own, and she never had surgery.

You can also pass this skill on to your children. At the end of my daughter Savannah's fifth birthday party, my son, Orion, was running and hit his head on a wagon, tearing the skin between his eyes. It was clear that he needed a few stitches. I calmly spoke to him as my close friend Kathryn and I headed to the emergency room at St. Vincent's Hospital here in New York City. He was seen by a great surgeon named Angel—Yes, Angel! I was able to talk Orion through the entire procedure, keeping him calm while he was getting stitches, relaxing his mind and his body. It was a profound moment between the two of us: I felt that we were very connected as I looked calmly and lovingly into his eyes. I saw that we trusted each other and knew everything would be ok. It was the beginning of my teaching him how to "play" with pain by relaxing into it, trusting himself and his body.

You are completely responsible for how you feel, what you think about, and how these feelings and thoughts impact your body. Knowing, owning, and using the tools that affect the mind-body connection lets you maintain or rebalance your emotional, mental, and physical states. Remember that every facet of this mind-body connection lives within you: it is all interconnected.

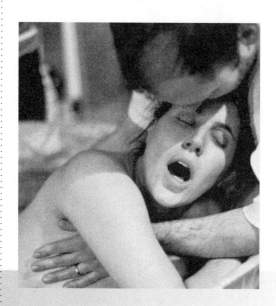

7 The Art and Science
of Labor and Birth

Your body is truly designed for childbirth in every way. If you can understand your body fully, which includes what goes on physiologically during childbirth, you'll have a more profound journey. This chapter will introduce you to the language and the physicality of each stage of labor and will show you how to bring your mind to each stage so that you progress as you intended.

Once you fully understand labor, you will be able to surrender to its expectations and power. When you can let go of your fears or concerns and replace them with knowledge, you will stop trying to control the birth and just let it happen. If you're harboring a fear of pain, however, the fear will come up during the childbirth, and your body won't be as pliable as necessary. The goal is to maintain control through knowledge, so that you don't have to control the moment.

What Has Already Happened

During your pregnancy, both your baby and your body have prepared for childbirth. Starting in the first trimester, your hormones allow the joints that hold the four bones of the pelvis together to stretch and loosen. By the ninth month, your pelvis has enlarged, and almost an inch of space has been added. Your uterus has changed as well. It has become a snug, rounded, hermetically sealed pouch; during labor, it will take on the shape of a funnel. Each contraction gently nudges the baby's head down through that funnel into the pelvis. At the same time that pressure numbs the lower half of your body, the pubic bone softens and spreads, and the vagina lubricates and stretches. The perineum, the diamond-shaped space just below the pelvic floor, becomes more elastic. Your body is designed to complete these movements without tearing. At this point, your body is ready for delivery.

The baby now takes up almost all of the room in the amniotic sac within your uterus. The best position for your baby to be in when you go into labor is head down, with the back of his head slightly toward the front of your tummy. When he passes into the bottom of your pelvis, he turns his head slightly so that the widest part of his head is in the widest part of your pelvis. The back of his head can then slip underneath your pubic bone, and, as he is born, his face sweeps across the perineum.

The baby's head is positioned right in front of the cervix, which is capped by a mucous plug that keeps the entire area clean and holds the cervix together. The top of the baby's head consists of softer tissue than the skull and is split into two fontanels that overlap during birth, allowing the head to pass through your vagina. It is a myth that the average baby's head is too big for a vaginal delivery.

What to Do If You Know Your Delivery Will Be Breech

A breech delivery occurs when baby's head is at the top of your uterus and the feet or the buttocks are presenting, instead of the head. Breech babies make up about 4 percent of all deliveries. There are several different positions that are all considered to be breech:

- Footling breech: feet first

- Complete breech: the baby is sitting on her heels (Buddha-style) or with her legs crossed (Indian-style)

- Frank breech: bottom first, with the feet up by the head

Mothers carrying breech babies might have heard that the "only" way they will be able to deliver a breech baby is to have a Cesarean. The truth is that there are several options for breech babies. The doctor or the midwife can turn the baby to a head-down position and proceed with a vaginal birth, he or she can perform a vaginal breech birth, or a doctor can perform a Cesarean birth.

If you know before the delivery that the baby is breech, however, there are several things you can do to help the baby turn. You can:

1. *Visualize the baby moving down,* with the head very deep in your pelvis, several times a day, especially in conjunction with the positions and the exercises listed in this list. You can also use your BornClear toolbox.

2. *Swim as often as possible.* This keeps your body and pelvis loose and relaxed. Swim in conjunction with doing a headstand in the water, if you have help.

3. *Do headstands with assistance, in a pool, as frequently as possible.* Don't do them if you're not in a pool, however; see the warning on page 132.

4. *Do pelvic tilts,* as recommended by the midwife Ina Mae Gaskin: Start as early as the eighth month, and lie in a tilted position on an inclined plane for ten minutes, twice a day. You could also lie on your back on the floor, with your knees flexed and your feet on the floor, with three large pillows placed under your bottom. Because gravity will then raise the baby up higher in the pelvis, some babies will just roll into the correct position. In one of Gaskin's studies, 89 percent of the babies spontaneously turned. You can also do this on an empty stomach with an ice pack on the top of your tummy, ten minutes twice a day. Or do the pelvic tilt in conjunction with music, visualization, or both.

5. *Play music for the baby.* Place your headphones inside your pants toward your pubic bone and play classical music for ten minutes six to eight times a day.

6. *Use a flashlight.* Shine the light through the skin on your belly, moving it slowly down from the top of the uterus toward your pubic bone, while you are in the tilted position.

7. *Massage your tummy.* Start with your left hand at the bottom of your abdomen and your right hand just above it. Move your hands clockwise around the right side of your tummy. As your right hand reaches the top of your abdomen, slide the left one over your right and move it down the left side of your tummy. Your left hand leads as you come full circle, continuing clockwise. Massage gently as if you are applying lotion. Massage for ten minutes or more, several times each day.

8. *Use a clothespin.* Place one on the small toe of each foot at the outside corner of the toenail, sideways, so that the toenail and the toe pad are stimulated for thirty minutes per day. This spot is considered a "moving down" acupressure point. You can also do this with finger pressure.

9. *Use a motion sickness band.* Place the band with the bead four finger widths above the inner ankle bone; this is another acupressure point that is used to stimulate the uterus. Do not use this point if you are experiencing preterm labor.

10. *Drink a glass of orange or another fruit juice.* After drinking your juice, lie down on your side, with your hips positioned higher than your feet. Babies move more after a sugar fix!

11. *Do the Cat-Cow asana.* Start on all fours with a flat back, then round your back and lift your head and buttocks toward the ceiling. End by returning to a flat back.

12. *Use the knee-chest position.* Lay down on your back on a mattress, and bring your hips up in a kneeling position. Your hips should be flexed slightly more than 90 degrees, with your thighs away from your tummy (not pressing against your tummy). Your head, shoulders, and upper back should lay flat on a mattress. Continue this position for fifteen minutes every two waking hours for five days.

13. *Do belly relaxing, followed by inversion.* Do this on an empty stomach. Have your partner place a shawl, a sheet, or a towel

under your hips as you lie on your back on the floor. Have your partner lift up on the corners of the cloth and shimmy you from side to side with very small movements, moving his hands to wiggle your belly from side to side. Do this for about five minutes. Then kneel at the top of a staircase, facing down the stairs. Walk your hands down two or three stairs into an all-fours position; have your partner stand in front of you to support your shoulders and balance you. Remain in this position for about five minutes or as long as is comfortable.

The following techniques to turn breech babies involve the assistance of a midwife, a specialist, or a medical professional:

14. *Try acupuncture.* Find an acupuncturist who is familiar with pregnancy and knows the points to stimulate to turn a breech baby.

15. *Try Webster's breech technique.* See a chiropractor who is experienced in this technique.

16. *Try the external version.* This can be done in the hospital at about thirty-seven weeks; see an ob-gyn for assistance and more information. It's done by applying pressure to your abdomen and manually manipulating the baby into a head-down position.

The Stages of Labor

The birth of your child is nothing less than an extraordinary feat of nature that involves an intricate sequence of events. Every pregnancy is different, and every childbirth is different. Yet most follow the same prescribed path of what physically unfolds in the body.

The Onset

The onset of labor is the official point at which labor begins. It marks the beginning of contractions or other signs that the baby is ready and your body is warming up. Think of it as an orchestra that is getting ready to play a symphony, and all of the sections are warming up and coordinating how to play in harmony together—the string instruments, the percussion section, and so on.

A variety of signals can indicate the onset of labor. They can include the breaking of the amniotic sac, the release of the mucus plug, or contractions or cramps that have a consistent pattern. If the amniotic sac ruptures, which is also called having your "water break," it can show up either like a slow leak or wetting your pants. It's not a gushing of water. Sometimes it is accompanied by a popping sound. Your water doesn't always break during the onset of labor. For my first child, my water didn't break until I actually gave birth.

When your mucus plug breaks, that is referred to as "bloody show." This will look like a thick, stringy, blood-tinged discharge. You may lose your mucus plug earlier than at the onset of labor. If you lose it during the onset of labor, however, there will be blood in it. You may also experience a backache, an upset stomach, or diarrhea. Some women report a sensation of warmth in the abdomen as labor begins.

If you feel that you have begun labor, you will want to connect with your doctor or midwife and tell him or her what you are experiencing to determine whether this is truly the onset and to set up your plan of communication from this point forward. I remember losing my mucus plug, and it had some blood in it on my underwear. It seemed like extra discharge, and I wasn't sure whether this was "it," so when I called my midwife, she confirmed that labor had begun.

The onset period can have a wide time span. Some people include this period within Stage 1 of labor, as we do here, but it is important to make the distinction so that we can dispel the misunderstanding and the "myth" of the fifty-hour labor. For example, when I lost my mucus plug with bloody show, I did not move into the next phase of early labor, where dilation began, until about forty hours later. Technically, however, I was in labor, but I was not experiencing pain. I felt the sensations of my body warming up for the delivery. I had some mild cramps, but I was completely able to walk around, go food shopping, and eat heartily (I remember having a yummy lamb curry stew). I also relaxed, watched a movie, and slept through the night. You may be able to do household chores, walk, take a bath, sleep, or gather your things if you are giving birth in a hospital or a birthing center. This is the time to nourish yourself and store up your energy.

So, when people tell you their birth stories and say that they were in labor for "fifty hours," they are not speaking responsibly. They are not differentiating the various phases of labor. Instead, they are unconsciously instilling fear in you. You might hear these stories and think that you will not be able to endure that amount of time. But the reality behind this conversation is very different. For me, the time from the onset of labor to giving birth to my child lasted a total of almost fifty hours: the first thirty-eight to forty hours were the onset, a comfortable warming-up period; Stage 1 was about nine hours of a mixture of easy, intense, and very intense sensations; Stage 2 lasted about three hours and was also a mixture of mild, intense, and powerful sensations; and Stage 3, comfortable and simple, lasted about thirty minutes.

Don't get attached to the possible time frames as you read through this section. I just want you to understand how long it may take for the baby to descend and be born, and how you will assist your body with your thoughts, emotions, spirit, and heart. So, as you get closer to your due date, don't watch your body as if you're waiting for a pot of water to boil. Try to relax, observe, and feel; let your labor unfold.

Stage 1: Early Labor into Active Labor

During early labor, pressure from the baby's head gradually stretches the tissue until it is paper-thin—a process known as "effacement." A small circular opening appears in the cervix, and each contraction widens it; this is called "dilation." Chapter 6 explained how the muscles of the uterus work, with the vertical muscles lifting up and over the top of the baby, nudging the baby down and out, as the horizontal muscles at the base of the cervix are effacing and dilating the cervix, allowing the baby to leave the uterus. These muscles work perfectly together during each contraction throughout each phase of Stage 1.

Early labor will end once the cervix opening has reached about three to four centimeters. By this time, the contractions/surges/cramps are about fifteen minutes apart, and there is now a consistent pattern or rhythm to the contractions while the cervix is dilating. The second phase of Stage 1 is when these surges are about eight minutes apart, and dilation is five to seven centimeters. The last stage is when you move into active labor. If you are giving birth at a birthing center or a hospital, you will normally leave your home during this phase, when you are about five centimeters dilated and the contractions are about two to five minutes apart and last for roughly sixty seconds each. When the cervix has dilated fully to ten centimeters in phase three, this is called "transition" inside of active labor.

As you move from the onset of labor to the initial phase of Stage 1, dilating a few centimeters, you will definitely feel a shift and will recognize that you are now in a different stage of labor. You may become quieter. You may no longer want food, and because the sensations now have a pattern, their intensity will increase.

Early in Stage 1, I was in the living room sitting with a couple of my very close friends. My partner and my midwife were on their way, and I started to feel the sensations. At one point I pulled out some paper, and my friend asked me to draw the contraction—what did it feel like? It was so great for me to connect with the sensations like that. We began timing the contractions and recording them on my drawings so that I could see the pattern while I experienced the feeling. This was a great meditation for me, as well as a distraction. Everyone became quieter, the lights were dimmed, and there was a beautiful fire roaring. I was calm and connected and felt intensity, excitement, nervousness, and fascination, all at the same time.

You can use whatever you need from the toolbox to make yourself comfortable. You may want to walk; rock on your birthing ball, if you have one; listen to music; do a visualization or have someone read you one; or simply rest. The more intense your sensations become, the more you will need to call on increased levels of endorphins and oxytocin. These chemicals will help you ease the sensations, begin to distort time, and close down your cerebral cortex, the thinking center in your brain. Use the tools to bring these chemicals on, so that you start to move into a quieter, more inward space.

Once you are in active labor, you'll feel the contractions getting longer, stronger, and closer together. You may not be able to discern a pattern to the contractions yourself, but your partner can help you record this information. At this point, you may just be dealing with your intense physical sensations, riding the physicality of the experience. You can try to visualize yourself opening, visualize the baby descending, or visualize the vertical and horizontal muscles gently supporting the baby's descent. Try all of these techniques in tandem, while you relax to the best of your ability, allowing your body to work and open.

You really cannot predict which tools you will use during labor, but I promise that you will know what to call on and what will work for you in this phase. It may be one of the visualizations, listening to soothing music, sitting on the edge of a birthing ball, rocking back and forth, taking a shower, placing hot compresses on your lower back or lower abdomen, sitting on the toilet, needing encouragement and reassurance from your partner or someone on your birthing team, or being massaged, touched, or held. Trust yourself to get to the place where you are feeling and not thinking. The chemicals being released in your body will guide you.

It may help if you hold yourself in certain specific positions during this stage of labor. Some that I have found to be most helpful are slow dancing (when you stand and hang onto your partner or doula), standing in a lunge position with a foot propped on a chair, sitting upright with a straight back, leaning back on to your partner or doula, rocking in a chair with your feet propped up, kneeling while you lean forward over the back of a chair, and lying on your back with your open knees to your chest as described earlier in the chapter. A birthing ball also provides other options. Each of these choices can be customized to fit your body.

Another tool you may use at this stage is your bond with your baby. Do not underestimate the power of your bond and communication with your baby. You can speak to him, both aloud and quietly in your mind, asking him to work his way downward and out of your body and gently nudging him with your thoughts and love. You may sense that your internal chemicals will allow your body to work in tandem with your intentions, guiding you and the baby. It is a team effort.

The transition phase typically marks the movement from Stage 1 into Stage 2; however, it can also include the last part of Stage 1, which can be the most intense. Many people experience nausea, involuntary shaking, or eliminating their bowels as their bodies begin to fully prepare for Stage 2. With my son, I remember throwing up at the end of Stage 1. It was so matter-of-fact, automatic, and simple; my body prompted me, and I realized I was "transitioning."

Stage 2: Birthing Your Baby

When you are fully dilated and your baby has descended into the birth canal, you are moving into Stage 2, birthing the baby. I want to dispel the myth of "the birth canal": some people think it is a long passage, but it is only your vagina, the length of your index finger.

It will be clear that you are moving into Stage 2, because you will feel different and will know it. Again, you may feel a bit of a pause or a break as you transition into Stage 2, or you might move actively into Stage 2 with the natural urge to push, as if you have to go to the bathroom. With each contraction, you will move your baby down the birth canal, after which the baby will soon "crown" (come through the vagina) to be born. The key is to take your time. In many respects, giving birth is like passing a hard bowel movement. Sometimes, you need privacy and some quiet time in order to eliminate. You instinctively know that once you relax your body, you will actually open naturally and then you can eliminate. The same is true for labor.

This stage can be as short as twenty minutes and as long as several hours. You are truly almost there. Use your mind to visualize your vagina opening and your baby coming toward you. Feel free to let him drift down on his own. You and your practitioner will sense how to "use" the contractions. Even though you will have the most natural urge to push, you may not want to force the baby out too quickly, which can increase your chances of tearing. Take your time; there is no rush. Notice whether you are holding your breath or clenching your jaw, and try to release all tension.

This stage always reminded me of when I learned how to scuba dive. The instructor said, "Remember, no matter what, don't hold your breath." The same is true with birthing. Use your breath, whatever breathing you feel will best support you now. Breathe through and with the contractions, breathing the baby down and out, breathing the vagina open. Use any of the breathing techniques in the toolbox.

When you continue to relax and not resist, you allow your chemicals to keep surging through your body, as they help you stay calm and work with your contractions. You might feel a natural "high," in which you remain clear and present. I remember this amazing stage when I used the contractions to ease the babies down and out—breathing with the contractions, using my Ujjayi breath. At one point during each childbirth, I could feel the baby's head come to the vagina as if the baby was ready to come through, but then the head would go back into the canal. This continued for a while, and I remember that it felt perfect and at the same time wild and exciting. Then the head reappeared for the last time about a quarter of the way through my vagina, and I put the palm of my hand down to feel the top of the baby's sweet head and beautiful soft hair. I was connecting with the baby for the first time outside of my body. I was so happy to be present and conscious at that moment and aware of the divinity of the experience. I felt clear and present, comfortable, and was talking to my midwife. I continued to use the contractions and push, and each of my two babies was born beautifully. First the baby's head came out, then the shoulders, and suddenly the rest of the small body slipped through. We were able to look directly into each other's eyes.

The tools that resonate most with you during pregnancy may not be the ones that you will use during birth. For example, when I gave birth to my daughter, Savannah, I was comfortable with all of the meditations and the visualizations, and I was happy to be surrounded by my family. During labor, however, all of a sudden I felt that I wanted to be totally alone. I went to the bathroom and locked the door. I knew that this was where I wanted to be, sitting in that position, in that environment, with that quietness. I sat on the toilet for what seemed like a little while, although it turned out to be almost an hour. Luckily, my mind was not working in real time. Sitting on the toilet felt good for me, and later I've heard that many women feel the same way. My feet were on the ground, but I was held up. Yet as I sat on the toilet, I was in intense pain, and I finally recognized that I was resisting the pain, holding on, holding my breath. I had an internal conversation with myself, and I talked myself into letting go, flowing with the pain. I knew the baby was at a bit of a standstill. I could feel that my muscles were locked, and the endorphins were definitely not present. I felt afraid and upset; the adrenaline was coming on. I knew that I needed to release endorphins so that the oxytocin would begin the contractions again, allowing the muscles to resume their work. I just sat with myself for a little while longer, and once I was able to let go of my fears, my body opened up. I felt a rush of hormones, the pain eased greatly, and I could feel my baby descending (all phases of Stage 1). I went from three centimeters to ten very quickly. I trusted, I allowed, and I surrendered—it was a very powerful experience. I was able to walk out of the bathroom and rejoin my partner and the midwife, knowing I was fully dilated. I was ready to head into the hot tub to quickly deliver the baby (the beginning of Stage 2). The pain, acting as my guide, encouraged my urge to push. I actually felt at ease and happy that I had let go and trusted myself, my body, my baby, my pain.

Trust your process, your tools, and your journey. They are uniquely yours. You may feel the need to use your voice to make sounds. This is a great release, so don't feel inhibited about how you may appear to others. Use and feel everything that you need to; making sounds can be another great tool and you can "ride" those releasing sounds to move through the next contraction. You may be surprised at what surfaces in your voice: it might sound very guttural, as if someone is lifting heavy weights. Whatever it is, do not judge it because no one else cares. Another of my BornClear clients, who had just delivered a few weeks earlier, told me what really had helped her in between contractions. Whenever she felt a very intense contraction, she told herself, "God wouldn't grant me something that I cannot handle."

When the baby is crowning and coming through the vagina, some women will experience a burning sensation called "the ring of fire." This feeling lasts for a very short time, maybe a few seconds. I felt the "ring of fire" for a few seconds with my first birth, and I didn't know what the heck it was. Then for my second birth I didn't feel it at all. As you can see, there are no hard-and-fast rules.

Stage 3: Birthing the Placenta

Stage 2 ends with the birth of your baby, but you still have more to do. Once you have given birth, there should be immediate skin-to-skin contact between you and your baby. During this time, the baby will still be attached to the umbilical cord. The third and final stage is birthing the placenta—this can take from twenty minutes to about an hour or so. At this point, you are still experiencing contractions as the placenta comes off the uterine walls. You will feel these contractions, but the birthing of the placenta is more of an automatic process. You may use some of the contractions to push out the placenta.

During this third and final stage, you might find that you are distracted, not really connected to the contractions because you are focused on your baby, your partner, and your feelings. You may also feel ready to begin breast-feeding at this time. If you are interested, take a look at the placenta when you birth it and see where your baby has lived and been nourished for the last nine months. Some people request to keep the placenta—many have done rituals around it or donated it to science. I asked for both of my children's placentas. We planted them under trees that we bought for each child. Those trees are growing big and strong to this day.

Issues That May Come Up During Labor

The following situations may arise as you proceed through each of the stages of labor. Being aware of everything that could occur in the birthing room will help you maintain your ideal birthing experience.

Dealing with a Stalled Situation

Labor can slow down, stall, or stop completely, in either Stage 1 or Stage 2. A stall during labor can occur for a variety of reasons, and, as I've said before, your mind-set may be one of them. Your fear, anxiety, or concern may have interrupted your focus. Your body analyzes this as a feeling of danger, sensing that you don't feel safe, and it releases catecholamines, which will trigger the "flight or flight" syndrome. These catecholamines immediately counteract the endorphins and the oxytocin, which are the chemicals that enable your contractions to progress. Once the flow of these chemicals shuts down, so does the labor.

Anxiety during labor is a completely natural reaction and is very common. Also, labor frequently slows down, stalls, or stops; it's completely normal. If this should happen to you, don't spin into deeper worries. The antidote is simply to trigger the release of more endorphins, which will then release oxytocin and restart the labor process. When you become deeply relaxed or regain a sense of safety, labor will begin again.

Some of the techniques you can use right away include visualizing your body opening and the baby descending. You can change whatever is distressing you about your environment—let your doula and/or your partner take on this mission. Other natural techniques include walking, taking a warm shower, or letting water run over you; water can be relaxing and it triggers endorphins. You can place hot towels or a hot water bottle on the base of your tummy or on the lower back; both are soothing and relaxing. You can also stimulate your erogenous zones, including your nipples, which will release oxytocin and endorphins. Some people use a breast pump to do this. You can also do it manually to yourself or have your partner do it for you. You will want to feel uninhibited with your birth team so that you can take advantage of this very effective option.

It is powerful to connect with and analyze what may have caused you to slow down, stall, or stop when you are right there in the moment. See if you can distinguish whether it was a physical, emotional, or mental issue. If a member of the hospital staff has interrupted you to express concerns and is continuing to upset you, have your doula or partner check in with that person. Make sure that the hospital staff frames their comments or suggestions in a positive context, so that they don't make you feel as if something is wrong, if that isn't the case. The main question to ask is whether the concerns are valid. You have every right to ask whether "the baby is in distress." If the answer is "no," then there really is nothing wrong. Remember that you can take as long as you need to re-center yourself and focus so that labor can progress. For example, you may be told that the baby's heartbeat is fluctuating. Don't let this alarm you: a baby's heartbeats can go really fast and then slow down. This is normal, but remember that the key question is "Is the baby in distress?"

My client Eva was faced with this exact scenario. Eva and her husband, Gary, believed that their doctor was pushing them toward having a C-section for a variety of nonmedical reasons. Their doctor kept implying that the birth was not going well and that "something was wrong," even though Eva, Gary, and the nurses around them knew that the baby was not in distress. Because Gary and Eva had a strong determination to deliver vaginally, they were able to ask their doctor the right questions (such as "Is the baby really in distress?") and stay in control. Gary protected Eva's space and ensured that she felt safe, quiet, and relaxed. Ultimately, Gary and Eva stood their ground, refocused on their context to create safety and relaxation, and were able to deliver their baby boy vaginally.

Postures and Positions for Birthing

If you do not have an epidural, you will be able to change your position during the second stage of labor. Practicing positions while you are pregnant may seem silly, but it will make them feel familiar when you really need them. This is another reason why it is important to master the information in this section as early in your pregnancy as possible. Many women find that using gravity, whether you are standing, sitting on the edge of a bed, sitting on a birthing stool, or squatting, can all help ease the baby down and out.

Propped sitting. Most mothers will be comfortable pushing if they are sitting up and slightly reclined back, and with their knees opened wide.

Standing, kneeling, or squatting. Some mothers may prefer to be more upright. Standing, kneeling, or squatting will allow you to swing your pelvis, moving the baby down. Squatting helps protect your perineum, making it less likely that you will tear or require the use of an episiotomy during your birth. In another position, called lap squatting, you dangle off the feet of your partner or doula: you are almost suspended in mid-air. You can also utilize a birthing stool which is low to the ground and supports you in a squatting position.

All fours. Some women find that going onto their hands and knees while they're in labor reduces pain. Many midwives recommend this position, since they believe it encourages the baby to shift into the best position faster. One study found that the women who went onto their hands and knees during delivery felt better and experienced less persistent back pain. If your baby is posterior or you are experiencing back pain, this position can be comforting. It allows your doula or partner to massage your back or apply counterpressure to help you be more comfortable.

Birthing ball. You can sit on a birthing ball during labor and then lean over a bed. This will allow you to sway your hips and lie down at the same time.

Instructions for a Water Birth

I believe that you should be encouraged to use a labor pool whenever you might find it helpful. It can be useful in both Stage 1 and Stage 2 of labor. If you choose to get into the water during early labor, however, before your contractions are strong and close together, the water may relax you significantly and may stop the labor altogether. That is why some practitioners limit the use of labor pools until labor patterns are established and the cervix is dilated to at least five centimeters.

Some women find a bath is useful during early labor for its calming effect and to determine whether labor has actually started. If contractions are strong and regular, no matter how dilated the cervix is, a bath could help you relax enough to facilitate dilation. Some practitioners suggest that the bath be used as a "trial of water" for at least one hour. Midwives have reported that some women can go from one centimeter to complete dilation within the first hour or two of immersion. The first hour of relaxation in the pool is usually the most effective and can often help you achieve complete dilation quickly.

If you have chosen to have a water birth, you can put yourself in any of the birthing positions discussed in the previous section while you are in the tub, depending on the water level. If you need to step out of the tub to enter these positions, make sure that you have a clean, dry area to work with.

Emergency C-Sections

Cesarean sections are an essential surgical procedure that can save the lives of women and babies when performed under some circumstances. But giving pregnant women the option of choosing to have a birth by C-section when it's not medically necessary is another matter entirely. Your obstetrician might suggest a C-section because of the convenience it provides for the doctor, as well as to quell his or her fear of litigation. In these cases, the doctor is putting his or her needs ahead of family values and your rights.

In his recent book *Born in the USA*, Dr. Marsden Wagner reports that the chances that an elective C-section will result in a woman's death are almost three times greater than in a vaginal birth. Women also face the risks that can accompany any major abdominal surgery—anaesthesia reactions and/or accidents, damage to blood vessels with massive hemorrhage, frequent infections, accidental extension of the uterine incision, damage to the bladder and the other abdominal organs, and internal scarring with adhesions, leading to painful bowel movements and painful sexual intercourse. The recovery time after a C-section is much longer than the recovery after a regular vaginal birth. What's more, babies born in elective C-sections are twice as likely to end up in neonatal intensive care and three times as likely to have serious pulmonary disorders in the newborn period compared to babies born in vaginal births.

I believe that the C-section rate in the United States has almost reached epidemic levels. Some of the promotion of C-sections relates to a present crisis in obstetrics, politics, and the health-insurance system in the United States. Through my BornClear class, I find that the American public is rapidly realizing that the high rate of C-sections in our country is a gigantic problem. However, this does not belie the fact that some C-sections occur out of medical necessity. If it is truly necessary, then a C-section is the perfect choice; and if you have a necessary C-section, you should not think that you "failed" at delivering your baby. At the same time, I do want to make clear that most women can and do have glitch-free natural births. You and your partner will need to be very clear about your intentions if you are presented with the option of a C-section. There is a difference between truly needing a C-section and electing an unnecessary C-section. You also need to understand, as Dr. Wagner explained in *Born in the USA*, that often "one intervention leads to another in a cascade of interventions that all lead to a C-section. An example of this cascade is an induction of labor with powerful drugs, which leads to increased labor pain, which leads to an epidural block to relieve the pain, which leads to slowing labor, which becomes 'failure to progress,' the number one diagnosis used to justify pulling the baby out with forceps or a vacuum extractor or performing C-section."

You should feel that your birth team has your best interest and health at heart and not their personal or professional agendas. Make sure that you fully verbalize your wishes and understand your practitioner's agendas and explanations, so that you can be fully responsible for all your choices and stay true to yourself. Having the freedom and the connection to pose these difficult questions to your birth team will lead you to the right choices for your ideal birth experience.

Dr. Jacques Moritz, the director of obstetrics at St. Luke's Hospital and Birthing Center, performs many Cesarean sections every year. From his experience, he believes that there are very few reasons for a truly emergency C-section. One would be an umbilical cord prolapse, in which the umbilical cord drops through the open cervix into the vagina ahead of the baby. The cord can then become trapped against the baby's body during delivery, preventing oxygen from reaching the baby. Another valid emergency would be if the baby's heart rate goes down and stays down for an extremely long period of time without coming up. This is another case where the baby is not getting oxygen.

The last scenario is placenta previa, when the placenta blocks the cervix and later detaches from the uterus, causing you to bleed vaginally. These are true emergencies because they happen without anyone's prior knowledge.

"However," said Dr. Moritz, "if you're pushing for four or five hours and the head is not coming down and it doesn't look like it is ever going to happen, you need a C-section. The word *emergency* shouldn't be used; you may just need a C-section."

Hospital deliveries, by nature, will end up with a higher Cesarean rate than at a birthing center or in a home birth with a midwife. Sometimes, the issue is timing—allowing the normal process to take its course no matter how long the baby and mother need. Dr. Moritz has told me that many hospitals simply will not allow you to push for hours on end to achieve a natural childbirth. Even so, if you are in a hospital, you need to know the difference between your doctor saying, "The baby is in distress, and the baby needs to come out soon," as opposed to telling you, "I'm ready to deliver this baby now, so we'll do it my way."

It is important to add that not every obstetrician is trying to promote C-sections. Dr. Wagner points to Jan Christilaw, a obstetrician, who commented on the rising C-section rate in the article "Too Posh to Push?" She wrote, "This [C-section] is a way of remedicalizing birth. I think birth is such an important cultural process that to divorce ourselves from its natural course is horrific."

Meet Elena

Elena was fully prepared for the childbirth she wanted. She worked with Angela Le, her acupuncturist, who was instrumental in her conceiving, and she followed the BornClear program. She worked on her relaxation exercises, took more time for herself, and made an effort to really connect with her partner. She made music CDs for the labor and constantly talked with the baby, played music for him, and kept a daily journal. She had all the right conversations with her doctor, who was understanding of her needs and in alignment with all of her intentions.

Even though Elena was about five days past her due date, she stayed true to her decisions. She heard what her doctor recommended but kept checking in with herself about what she really felt. She reminded herself that she could have what she wanted—a peaceful loving birth for her and the baby and her partner. She held onto that positive mind-set, getting support from Angela, me, and her partner, Ali.

The doctor was pushing her to schedule a C-section. Elena wanted to plug along, however, and she labored for a long time naturally, resisting the idea. Yet everything she had planned on a concrete level did not turn out as expected once she started her labor. Elena did not plan to take medication—then she opted for Pitocin. She did not want an epidural but asked for one anyway. In the end she acquiesced to having a C-section, even though she knew that she could not hold or nurse her new baby boy right away.

After the birth, the doctor told Elena that the baby's umbilical cord was about a third of the length it should have been. Then Elena realized how smart the baby had been not to come out—he knew. Elena trusted the intelligence of her baby and the brilliance and intelligence of our bodies and the universe. This is how she peacefully resolved having a C-section.

Elena learned more than a few lessons from the whole experience. First, she realized that not only was it important to communicate what you need and want, but you also have to allow things to unfold and trust that there is a reason for everything. She also learned that there is a difference between knowing what you want and being really attached to it. In the end, Elena had to let go of her idea that a perfect birth could only be a natural vaginal birth. In the end, she was happy to have a healthy baby boy, no matter how he had been birthed.

Other Procedures to Be Aware Of

The following are a variety of medical practices that you need to be knowledgeable about, for your sake and the baby's. Make sure that you fully understand each procedure to determine whether they fit into your current context for this birth.

Episiotomy. An episiotomy is a surgical incision that is made to enlarge the vagina. A small incision is usually made while the mother is under a local anaesthetic, and the incision is closed after the baby's delivery. Many doctors perform episiotomies because they believe that these will lessen perineal trauma, minimize postpartum pelvic floor dysfunction, reduce the loss of blood at delivery, and protect against neonatal trauma. It has also been noted, however, that episiotomies actually cause all of these problems. In fact, episiotomies have been shown to be the principal risk factor for severe tearing during delivery, which is the injury that they are supposed to prevent. An episiotomy is also a major risk for infection, incontinence, hemorrhage, and, for some women, loss of sexual pleasure. Women who have episiotomies take longer to heal from delivery, even when compared to women who have equivalent tears.

In 1995, a review of the best episiotomy research by the Cochrane Library (a frequently updated, highly respected electronic library of reviews of the scientific evidence on different obstetric practices) found that when done routinely, the procedure increases the trauma and complications of birth. The general consensus now among perinatal scientists and obstetricians is that the ideal rate of episiotomy is 5 to 10 percent of all vaginal births. Episiotomies should be done only in urgent situations, such as cases of fetal distress due to a compressed umbilical cord that require a hasty vacuum extraction.

While you are pregnant, you can work on preventing the need for an episiotomy by doing the following: Practice daily squats to increase the flexibility of your perineal muscles and skin. Eat foods that are rich in vitamins E, C, and A. You can also try frequent perineal massages with olive oil or an oil of your choice during pregnancy, as well as practice the Kegel exercises that are listed in the toolbox.

During delivery, you can avoid an episiotomy by abstaining from pain medication, so that you can feel when to stop pushing. Choose a birthing position in which you are not lying on your back, because that would slow the baby's delivery once his or her head is crowning.

Hot water bottles or hot compresses during Stage 2 may also help. Your doctor or midwife might know how to lift the baby out over the perineum and can instruct you on how to breathe properly between contractions so that an episiotomy is not necessary. When I was birthing my daughter, I had a very slight tear that healed in a few days, and with my son, my second birth, there was no tear at all.

Circumcision. A boy has a hood of skin, called the foreskin, that covers the head of the penis. In circumcision, the foreskin is removed from the glans, exposing the end of the penis. The foreskin is first slit lengthwise so that the circumcision instrument can be inserted, and then the foreskin is cut off. Approximately 56 percent of all newborn boys—about 1.1 million babies—are circumcised in the United States each year. In recent years, the rate of uncircumcised boys in the United States has increased. Parents who choose circumcision usually cite religious beliefs, concerns about hygiene, or cultural or social reasons, such as the desire to have a son look like the other men in the family.

The foreskin makes up as much as half or more of the penile skin system and has three known functions: protective, sensory, and sexual. During infancy, the foreskin is attached to the glans and protects it from urine, feces, and abrasion from diapers. According to the American Academy of Pediatrics, "The foreskin protects the glans throughout life." It also keeps the glans soft and moist and shields it from trauma and injury. Without this protection, the glans can become dry, calloused, and desensitized from exposure and chafing. The foreskin may have other functions that are not yet recognized or understood.

Uncircumcised boys can learn how to clean beneath the foreskin once the foreskin becomes retractable (which usually occurs sometime before age five). Poor hygiene can impact both uncircumcised and circumcised boys. If you choose not to have your son circumcised, talk to your pediatrician about the proper way to keep the penis clean.

Circumcision also carries potential risks. First, it is a surgical procedure, and complications such as minor bleeding and local infection can occur, although they are rare. Second, the procedure is painful and can be traumatic. Most doctors will now provide anesthesia, as either a topical cream or an injectable anesthetic. Some circumcised males suffer from scarring, skin tags, or a curvature of the penis, which may be linked to difficulty in ejaculating later in life. A number of studies have found that there is a loss of sensitivity in the glans after circumcision, and other studies show that many uncircumcised men report having more sexual, sensual sensations than circumcised men have. It is a very personal decision. If you decide on circumcision, it should be performed within the first two to three weeks after birth. A pediatrician, a family doctor, or an obstetrician can perform the procedure. In some instances, doctors may decide to delay the procedure (in the case of premature babies) or forgo it altogether, such as if there are physical abnormalities of the penis.

Vitamin K. Newborn infants routinely receive a vitamin K shot after birth, in order to prevent (or slow) a rare problem of bleeding into the brain that occurs weeks after birth in one out of ten thousand babies. Vitamin K promotes blood clotting. The fetus has low levels of vitamin K, as well as other factors that are needed in clotting. The body maintains these levels very precisely. For preventive measures, newborns have been receiving vitamin K routinely since the 1960s. Traditionally, vitamin K has been given as a shot. Studies show that vitamin K given orally, however, is just as effective and possibly a better solution.

Some mothers supplement their diets with foods that are high in vitamin K—such as spinach, broccoli, brussels sprouts, cauliflower, and watercress—prior to childbirth and in the postpartum period. Nursing mothers can take vitamin K supplements to support the baby as well. In some states the vitamin K shot is presented as compulsory. If so, you need to understand the procedure, and see if there may be flexibility on administering the shot, depending on what you resolve for yourself and your child.

Vacuum extraction. During Stage 2, a suction device may be placed on the baby's head, which a doctor uses to pull during contractions to assist the speed of birth. A doctor may suggest using a suction device if medications have reduced your pushing effectiveness, if the baby's size or position is slowing delivery, or if fetal distress is suspected.

You can avoid vacuum extraction by not having an epidural, which has been shown to be associated with an increased need for assistance. This is partly because your pushing efforts are less effective when you cannot feel what you are doing. If epidural anesthesia is needed, many midwives and doctors believe that the mother's pushing efforts will be more effective if she is allowed to rest without pushing actively until the baby's head is very low in the pelvis, allowing the force of the contractions alone to do much of the work before the mother begins to actively assist the birth.

Forceps. Forceps are a pair of steel instruments that look like two long handles that are each attached to a spoon. They are placed in the vagina on either side of baby's head and then locked together. During Stage 2, the doctor will use the forceps to help tug the baby out during contractions to assist or speed birth. A doctor may suggest using forceps if medications have reduced your pushing effectiveness, if the baby is high in the birth canal, or if fetal distress is suspected.

You now understand the physical path of birth and all of the ways that you can use the methods in the toolbox to assist you. As your context continues to take shape, think about and visualize what you really want for this birth. Feel yourself moving through all of the stages without being attached to issues of timing or exactly how the childbirth will look; instead, concentrate on how you want it to feel—intellect merging with intuition.

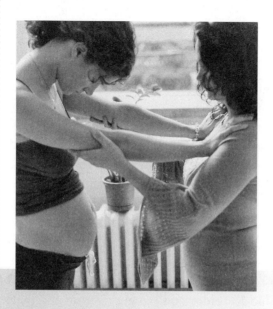

8 The Birth Plan: The Art of Creating Alignment

All your planning and practicing with the toolbox have brought you closer to fulfilling your context for your birth. The next level of planning allows you to verbalize your context, including the details and the logistics that this birth will entail, and to align with all of the people involved. The point of this exercise is to make sure that everything related to the birth is discussed and all of your questions are answered.

The best way to achieve this is with a written document called a birth plan. Creating this document allows you to uncover aspects about this birth that you may not have thought of, and it could require some emotionally deep decision making on your part. I have found that most women who have birthing "horror stories" were never really physically, emotionally, or mentally prepared for their childbirths. These women neglected this deep level of preparation, which could have contributed to a greater understanding of the birthing process. Their new knowledge would have enabled them to clearly envision the childbirth and then relax and trust the process. They did not take the time, or perhaps were emotionally unable, to have all of the necessary conversations with their partners or birth teams, which would have resulted in mutually agreed-on plans for how various aspects of the birth would be dealt with.

You'll find that this kind of preparation will preempt unnecessary surprises, breakdowns, anxiety, or even medical interventions during birth, all of which can lead to an unfulfilling or, worse, disappointing experience. The birth plan allows you to see where you have limited yourself, and gives you the opportunity to address all of your needs and wants and to understand your practitioner's philosophies, personality, and procedures more deeply.

There are two important aspects of the birth plan. First, you will craft a document that identifies each of your wishes for the birth. Then, you will gather together and align a birth team that will share and implement your vision. These two actions will help you create "alignments" for yourself and everyone around you. In this way, you will be able to share your singular vision, one that puts you at ease and empties your mind of all mental and emotional clutter and distractions. As a result, you will have the power to focus on yourself and your baby during the childbirth experience.

The Beauty of Creating Alignment

In the BornClear philosophy, *alignment* means an understanding that everyone involved is united and clear on a particular way of thinking, a specific objective, or both. The alignment process is successful when everyone can communicate directly and honestly about his or her thoughts, questions, and concerns and in the end reach agreement. Best of all, alignment will give you the opportunity to find your voice: the ability to ask for whatever you want or need. To me, finding and fully expressing one's voice is freedom.

Each alignment conversation allows you to understand your partner and your medical practitioner(s), as well as their beliefs and practices.

Without it, the hospital, the birthing center, or the midwife's staff would follow their usual prescribed routines, which may or may not be exactly what you want. By having these conversations, you are allowing yourself the opportunity to make requests that will help you fulfill your context.

Alignment begins when you become a clear, powerful communicator. One aspect of this skill is conveyed in your tone. A calm tone can facilitate any conversation so that others can digest and hear it more easily. When you start an alignment conversation, try to be sensitive to your tone. Notice whether you are calm, clear, and present, or whether you get triggered into reacting to something that upsets you. This level of self-awareness and consciousness takes discipline, but it is deeply satisfying to master the beauty of communication.

How do you create alignment? One way is to make sure that others fully understand your intentions. One type of communication that I find to be particularly effective is called "active listening" or "mirroring back." When you are talking with someone and sharing information, ask the person to repeat back to you what he or she heard. From this vantage point, you can see whether you have spoken clearly and addressed your issues accurately or whether the person missed any part of your communication. Mirroring conversations gives you the opportunity to be thorough and not assume that the person you are speaking with knows what you meant or heard you completely. Instead, you can see for yourself what you failed to communicate. By also mirroring the other person's conversation back to him or her, you are showing your commitment to be heard and understood, as well as your commitment to hear and understand that person. This technique is a powerful life tool—it holds you fully accountable for speaking in such a way that you are heard and for listening skillfully so that issues get resolved.

Most people get stuck in their own heads with their own ideas or thoughts, because they want to make their points heard. Or they are so distracted by their own thinking that they cannot listen to others. This is when miscommunications or arguments occur. The key is not to give up when you know that a topic or an issue is still not agreed upon or understood, or alignment is not yet complete. If you truly listen to each other, even if you don't agree, at least you each will gain a better understanding of the other person.

You also need the courage to ask tough questions, even if you think you might sound foolish. Stop judging yourself or taking things personally, and be willing to have conversations that are powerful and necessary. These difficult conversations can allow you to release pent-up conflicts that cause stress in your relationships.

Dispelling and clarifying all assumptions will leave every relationship in the clearest state possible. When we assume, we may think that our interpretations are true before we ever check in with others to clarify what they really mean. Fear, embarrassment, judgment, or a lack of compassion can allow you to believe in the truth of your assumptions, regardless of the facts. It is always better to ask questions than to make an assumption, because assumptions set us up for suffering.

If you end up mumbling to yourself about something after an alignment conversation, this is a sign that you are still not completely clear about the issue. Make sure that you address this topic again, and get the other person to agree on it at the next opportunity. Your mumbling hints at a fear or an intuition that something was left unresolved; either way, don't let it slide without addressing it fully. If you don't deal with it, the issue will never go away. Worse, your dissatisfaction will manifest in countless ways, such as blame or other types of destructive behavior.

When you have addressed everything you need with this level of honesty, you will have complete peace of mind. You'll feel even more connected, safe, and taken care of by your partner and your team. Completing this process makes you fully responsible for your context, leaving you empowered. Afterward, you can relax, knowing that you did your best to express and take care of your desires.

Addressing Your Birth Plan

These seven steps provide a road map for how to work with your birth plan:

1. Confirm your context (your list of desires) in writing with your partner. This will be your mission statement for the birth. Add any of your own statements to this wish list as well:

I would like my birth to be (add your adjectives here).

I am planning to deliver my baby at _____.

I would like a (doctor, doula, midwife) *to be present at the birth.*

Others who will be present include _____.

2. Review all of the possible procedures and practices: use the following list of suggestions and write down the ones that positively resonate with you. For example, instead of writing, "Would you like to use a wheelchair, if it's available, or walk to the room?" you would write, "I would (or would not) like to use a wheelchair, if it's available." You'll find that as you go through this list, you'll make some important decisions. Reference your wishes and your context to these decisions.

   For example, if you desire a hospital birth that is quiet, peaceful, and private, your birth plan should suggest ways to implement these ideas, such as requesting limited fetal monitoring, which is less distracting than constant monitoring. Or you could put a sign on the door to your hospital room that reads, "Enter quietly." These small steps can allow other people whom you will be in contact with during the birth to be sensitive to your wishes before they enter.

3. Make a list of open questions and issues you still have, and be prepared to share all of this with your medical practitioner during an alignment conversation. If you are using a doula and/or are having a family member or a friend attend your childbirth, make sure you set up alignment meetings with each of them.

4. If you are giving birth in a birthing center or a hospital, it would be beneficial to do a tour of the facility before you have the alignment conversation with your practitioner. Write down whatever questions you have, based on what you saw, including any concerns that have come up.

5. Set up a meeting with your medical practitioner for an alignment conversation. During this conversation, review your context with your practitioner. Make sure you cover all of your questions,

your wishes, and the desired mood for your childbirth. Address all of your concerns, and do not end the conversation until everything is completely clear for you and your team. Ask your practitioner whether there is anything you have not asked or addressed or should know. You should feel excited after having this conversation, knowing that your team is aligned and everything is agreed upon.

6. When you have time to yourself, reexamine your conversations to make sure that you have addressed everything. If you still have any concerns, questions, or fears that you are mumbling about to yourself, schedule another appointment to get these issues addressed and resolved.

7. Make up a simple one- or two-page summary of all that you and your team have agreed on. This will be your final birth plan. Everyone involved with your childbirth should have a copy. Give a copy of the plan to your practitioner to keep in his or her file, and bring a few copies along to the birth to give out to those present from your birth team. If you are giving birth at a hospital or a birthing center, you may want to have a copy of the birth plan taped to the door of your room, as well as having extra copies available for other people who may be supporting you who are not on your immediate birth team. At this point, you should feel confident that this childbirth is under your direction.

Here is a list of all of the possible scenarios, procedures, and details that may occur during your childbirth. These conversation starters provide the framework for you to create alignment conversations with others.

Hospital or Birthing Center: First Stage of Labor

- What are all of the procedures and the necessary paperwork for admission that can be completed beforehand?
- Would you like to use a wheelchair, if it's available, or walk to the room?

- How do you feel about having a routine IV prep on admission, if that is part of the automatic procedures? What are your choices?

- Do you want to return home until labor progresses further, if an examination reveals that you are fewer than four centimeters dilated and other factors do not warrant admission?

- Do you want a private birthing room if it's available?

- Do you want subdued lighting and drawn drapes?

- Would you like to bring music to the hospital or the birthing center? (If so, make sure there is an electrical outlet available or that your player has proper batteries.) What music would you like to bring?

- Do you want to have an enema for bowel elimination?

- Do you want to have a vaginal shave or clipping?

- Do you want pictures or a video taken—and by whom?

- Do you want telephone inquiries relayed to the birthing room?

- Would you like to limit visits only to the necessary hospital staff?

- Would you like the staff around you to refrain from making references to "pain" or "hard labor"?

- Would you like the staff to be as quiet as possible?

- Would you like and can you have a sign on the door stating, "Please enter quietly"?

- Do you want your partner or birthing companion to be present at all times?

- Do you prefer to be free of the blood pressure cuff between readings?

- Would you like a continuous electronic fetal monitor (EFM) or only if it is medically necessary?

- Does the hospital or the birthing center have a soft spandex tube for securing EFM monitors?

- Would you like to discontinue the EFM once a pattern is established and then switch to intermittent monitoring of the baby's heart with a fetoscope?

- If there is no fetal distress, would you like *no* EFM at all?
- Would you like to make the initial suggestion for anesthetics (epidural) or analgesics?
- Would you like your doctor or midwife to recommend when anesthetics (epidural) or analgesics seem appropriate?
- If labor is prolonged, would you like to have a light snack? (You may want to consider bringing in your own favorite snacks.)
- Would you like fluids and light food, including juices, herbal tea, broth, toast, and crackers? Ice chips and popsicles?
- Would you like the freedom to walk or move during labor?
- Would you like the freedom to change positions and assume labor positions of your choice?
- Would you like the minimum or the maximum number of vaginal exams?
- When would you consent to any augmentation of labor, including drugs (Pitocin, stripping of membranes, and so on)?
- Will you want to allow labor to take its natural course without others making references to "moving things along"?
- Will you want to practice natural oxytocin stimulation, including nipple or clitoral stimulation, in the event of stalled or slow labor?
- Will you want uninterrupted privacy to perform natural oxytocin stimulation?
- Would you like for you and your birth team to be fully apprised and consulted before the introduction of any medical procedure?
- Would you like a labor tub or shower? (If so, make sure that the hospital or birthing center has a chair or a stool you can bring into the shower with you.)
- Would you like to use a birthing ball?

Home Birth: First Stage of Labor

- Do you want subdued lights and drawn drapes?
- Would you like to play music?

- Do you want pictures or a video taken—and by whom?
- Which supplies will you need to get for your home birth, where should you order them from, and where will you store them?
- Would you like the midwife and the doula to be as quiet as possible?
- Do you want your partner or birthing companion to be present at all times?
- Would you like your midwife to recommend when to use various pain inhibitors—hot compresses, and so on?
- If labor is prolonged, would you like to have a light snack? What would you like to eat?
- Would you like fluids and light food, such as juices, herbal tea, broth, toast, crackers, your favorite foods, and snacks? Ice chips and popsicles?
- Would you like the minimum or the maximum number of vaginal exams?
- When would you consent to any augmentation of labor (stripping of membranes, and so on)?
- Will you want to practice natural oxytocin stimulation, including nipple or clitoral stimulation, in the event of stalled or slow labor?
- Will you want uninterrupted privacy to perform natural oxytocin stimulation?
- Would you like a labor tub or shower?
- Would you like to use a birthing ball?

Hospital or Birthing Center: Second Stage of Labor

- Would you like to request letting your natural birthing instincts facilitate the descent of the baby, with mother-directed breathing until the crowning takes place?
- Would you like to remain in the tub for water birthing, if this is available?
- What is the hospital's or the birthing center's rate of episiotomy? Is this medical facility's staff willing to be aligned with my intentions on episiotomy, circumcision, bonding with the

baby at birth, and the procedures for the baby that are in my current birth plan?

- Would you like the doctor or midwife to inform you before performing an episiotomy?
- If an episiotomy is necessary, would you like a topical anesthetic?
- Would you like to be able to request the birthing position of your choice?
- Would you like the use of the birthing stool or a bed for birthing in a squatting position?
- Would you like the use of a suctioning device, rather than forceps, if assistance is medically necessary?
- Would you like to determine for yourself whether you would like assistance?
- Would you like the use of a mirror to enable you to see the crowning and the birth?
- How do you feel about other children being present at birth, if this applies?
- How do you feel about other children being present shortly after labor, if this applies?
- Will the partner/doula/nurse/doctor/midwife "catch" the baby?
- Who will announce the sex of the baby?
- Do you prefer immediate skin-to-skin contact, with the baby being placed on your stomach? Can your partner also join in this?
- Would you prefer your partner or birthing companion to remain with you in the operating room and the recovery room in the event of a C-section?
- Will your partner hold the baby after the C-section delivery and accompany the baby to the nursery or another room?
- Do you prefer to allow at least thirty to forty minutes for a natural placenta delivery?
- Do you prefer immediate breast-feeding to assist in natural placenta expulsion?

- Would you like a uterine massage every fifteen minutes and nipple stimulation to assist the placenta birth, if needed?

- Would you like to limit cord traction, Pitocin, or the manual removal of the placenta unless in an emergency?

Home Birth: Second Stage of Labor

- Would you like to remain in the tub for water birthing?

- How do you feel about an episiotomy versus tearing? Would you like the midwife to inform you before doing an episiotomy?

- If an episiotomy is necessary, would you like a topical anesthetic?

- Would you like to determine for yourself whether you would like assistance?

- Would you like the use of a mirror to enable you to see the crowning and the birth?

- If you have other children, how do you feel about them being present at the birth?

- If you have other children, how do you feel about them being present shortly after labor?

- Will the partner/doula/midwife "catch" the baby?

- Who will announce the sex of the baby?

- Do you prefer immediate skin-to-skin contact, with the baby being placed on your stomach? Can your partner also join in this?

- Do you have a backup procedure in place, should you need to get to a hospital?

- Would you like a uterine massage every fifteen minutes and nipple stimulation to assist a placenta birth, if needed?

After the Birth: Hospital or Birthing Center

- Would you like the use of bright lights to be temporarily halted for the first hour after birth?

- Would you like to allow the vernix to be absorbed into the baby's skin and to delay "cleaning or rubbing"? (The vernix is the waxy white substance that is found coating the skin of newborns. It is the oil of the baby's skin, coupled with the cells that have sloughed off in the womb. Some people believe that it has antibacterial properties. To remove the vernix, you can request the use of a soft cloth.)

- Would you like the cord to be clamped and cut only after pulsation has ceased?

- Whom would you like to cut the cord?

- Would you like your baby to remain with you for one hour after delivery?

- What is the course of events after this point?

- Do you care to delay or eliminate the use of erythromycin or other salves for the baby's eyes to allow optimal sight for bonding?

- Would you prefer to have oral vitamin K to be used, if it is available, rather than an injection?

- Would you prefer not to have vitamin K administered at all?

- Would you like a soft cloth or blanket placed between the baby and the scale?

- How do you feel about circumcision? When will this be performed?

- Where will your partner be sleeping during your hospital stay?

- Would you like to have the baby's footprints made for the baby's birth book?

- Do you prefer to breast-feed several times during the first few hours of the baby's life?

- Would you like to request that there be only breast-feeding—no bottles, formula, pacifier, or artificial nipples?

- Can the hospital or the birthing center supply you with a peri-bottle to use for your perineum when you urinate and cold packs for your perineum that you would wear in your underwear for healing and soothing?

After the Birth: Home Birth

- Would you like to allow the vernix to be absorbed into the baby's skin and to delay "cleaning" or "rubbing"? (The vernix is the waxy white substance that is found coating the skin of newborns. It is the oil of the baby's skin, coupled with the cells that have sloughed off in the womb. Some people believe that it has antibacterial properties. To remove the vernix, you can request the use of a soft cloth.)

- Would you like the cord to be clamped and cut only after pulsation has ceased?

- Whom would you like to cut the cord?

- Do you care to delay or eliminate the use of erythromycin or other salves for the baby's eyes, to allow optimal sight for bonding?

- Would you prefer to have vitamin K administered to the baby?

- How do you feel about circumcision? When will this be performed?

- Would you like to have the baby's footprints made for the baby's birth book?

- Are you committed only to breast-feeding—no bottles, formula, pacifier, or artificial nipples?

Conversations with Your Birth Team

It is so important that you feel that your team is made up of people who consider themselves partners in this birth. Your birth team will include your partner, your medical practitioner and his or her medical team, and even friends who will be with you when you are laboring and birthing. You will also have an extended birth team that can include friends and family members who will be around you when you are birthing but not actually present at the birth. You want to be clear with each member of your team(s), telling them what you want from them physically, emotionally, or spiritually. You will need to have all of the necessary conversations with them to make sure that they are aligned with, and supportive of, your wishes.

Make a list of all of the people whom you need to have conversations with. This should include everyone who will share your context. You may want to make requests of people who will have to put aside their own opinions of your context in order to support you. You may also need to address certain concerns you have with specific friends or family members. For example, many of my clients have felt stressed by expectations or requests from their parents or in-laws to be included in the childbirth or to help afterward. If you feel this kind of pressure, I recommend that you look at your context. Determine what you really need and want from these people and communicate exactly that. Use the alignment process described previously, and set up times to have these conversations.

Questions to Ask Your Birth Team(s)

- Do you fully understand my context for this birth?
- Can you support my family and this context when I need you to?
- Do you have a clear idea of the flow and the intrinsic procedures and protocols of the hospital, of the birthing center, or during a home birth? How long have you been associated with this particular facility?
- When will you arrive at the home/hospital/birthing center?
- What are your thoughts about induction of labor?
- Let's decide and discuss who will be accountable for what, besides the midwife or the doctor.

Touring Your Birth Facility

Once you have chosen a medical practitioner, you will need to investigate the hospital or the birthing centers he or she is affiliated with, if you don't choose a home birth. It is very common to take a tour of the hospital or the birthing center. Determine how long it will take to get from your home to the birthing location, factoring in traffic and weather. Be sure to have an alternate route in mind in case your first route isn't possible. If you are not driving and need to arrange for someone on your birth team to drive you to the facility, set up those plans at least three weeks before your due date.

As you look around the hospital or the birthing center, see whether these spaces are in keeping with your context. Bring your working birth plan with you, and use it to ask questions of the staff. If their policies are not aligned with your intentions, then you might want to consider a different hospital or birthing center. This may mean that you will need to choose another medical practitioner as well.

When my client Sherry went through all of the dimensions of the BornClear course, including the alignment conversations, she realized that she felt an uncomfortable nagging feeling she could not shake. She was definitely mumbling to herself, and she knew in her heart that even though she was okay with her practitioner, she did not feel safe in the birthing facility that she chose. She changed her birthing team about a month before her due date and was so happy that she did. She felt relieved and at peace and gave birth to a beautiful baby girl as she had intended. The message here is, trust your intuition!

Be sure to address these additional questions during your tour of the facility:

- Does this facility have a pre-admission policy so that I can fill out all of the paperwork before my due date?
- What types of birthing rooms are available?
- Is there a tub I can use during labor, delivery, or both?
- What procedures during the birth are standard or routine?
- How many support people are allowed in the room?
- What are the standard procedures for the newborn?
- Is this facility breast-feeding friendly?
- Are its lactation consultants on staff?
- Can cameras, video cameras, and tape recorders be used?
- Can I play music in my room during delivery?
- Where is the best place to park, day or night?
- What is the best entrance to use, day or night?

Pre-Planning a Home Birth

- Do a walk-through of your home with your midwife and anyone else who is on your team. Make sure that you identify where supplies will be kept, as well as possible tools for the birth. The doula, the midwife, or both, should know where the bathrooms, the bedrooms, the showers, the tubs, and the hot tubs are located.

- Does your midwife have standard procedures during a birth?

- How many support people will the midwife allow in the room?

- What are her standard procedures for the newborn?

- Create a checklist for supplies that you will need to provide.

- Order all of the supplies for a home birth. See the Resources section at the end of this book.

- Make sure that you and your midwife have a clear plan for a backup doctor, and meet with that doctor at least one month before the due date.

What Happens When Things Don't Go Your Way

As in all aspects of life, there are no guarantees that your childbirth will go as you've planned. Although this level of detailed planning and mental and emotional preparation allows for few surprises, no one can foresee the future, and not everything may end up going your way. For example, there is no guarantee that interruptions in a hospital or a birthing center won't happen, despite your best attempts to keep them to a minimum. The beauty of your preparation is that it will allow your partner and birth team to support you when surprises arise—they will do a good job of protecting and ensuring your context. In this way, you will be supported in handling whatever comes your way during the birth.

Meet Eva

Eva is one of my favorite clients, and not because her birth went exactly as she expected. In fact, it couldn't have gone more differently. Yet she was able to stay true to her context because she did the work in advance and managed to stay calm and mentally flexible. Eva engaged her husband, Gary, in helping her design how she wanted their childbirth to proceed. She taught him to guide and coach her through the labor. During the pregnancy, they did the toolbox exercises together, and both gained confidence for the experience to come. By using the fear-eliminating exercise and repeatedly visualizing a perfect birth, Eva went from a state of fear and apprehension to feeling, as she said, "really and truly peaceful and happy and ready and, most of all, confident in the birthing to come. As I neared my due date, people asked me whether I was nervous, and I could honestly say, 'No, I'm ready.'"

The last weeks of her pregnancy were very difficult, primarily because her due date came and went. Eva and Gary found themselves at odds with their doctor, who seemed anxious to induce. Eva became increasingly stressed and was disappointed because her delivery was not exactly following her birth plan, in which she had been clear that she did not want labor to be induced. The night before her scheduled induction, however, Eva went into labor and delivered a healthy baby boy.

"I owe the outcome—a perfect labor—to education and confidence," Eva said. "I educated myself by reading and talking to people so I had the knowledge necessary to understand the processes of labor. I gained confidence in my ability, not just to birth, but to make decisions about the birth, with Denise's guidance. The many visualizations, fear-elimination exercises, practice sessions, and conversations with my husband put me in a place where I knew without a doubt that I could do it. With education, a plan, and a good state of mind, I know now that you can get through any obstacle. If you can see the result in your mind and feel confident in your ability to achieve it, you will."

Packing Your Bag

Have your overnight suitcase or "birth bag" packed during the third trimester if you are going to give birth in a hospital or a birthing center. Inside will be everything you will need for yourself, your partner, and the baby. Remember to pack for "just in case" situations: if you or the baby has to stay in the hospital longer than the traditional few days.

If you are having a home birth, make sure you have baby supplies handy: a hat, outfits for the baby, golden seal powder to heal the umbilical cord, receiving blankets, warm items if needed, gentle baby wipes, and a baby book for footprints.

Your birth bag should include:

- Important paperwork. Bring at least four copies of your birth plan, so that you can tape one on the door and hand out the rest to others on your team, including staff and nurses. Also included in this paperwork are your hospital registration, insurance card, any necessary prenatal reports, and a large envelope to bring home documentation, such as discharge papers and other important medical information.

- Soft, comfortable clothes that have easy frontal access for breast-feeding. Also bring nightgowns, a bathrobe, slippers, socks, hair ties, several changes of underwear, and bras (nursing bras).

- All of your BornClear tools—audio recordings of your favorite visualizations, oils, candles, music, headphones, your MP3 player, a birthing ball (if the hospital or birthing center does not have one), CDs, aromatherapy items, a night light, hot water bottles, and hot compresses.

- Snacks, including your favorite drinks and foods, lollipops, and change for vending machines.

- An extra pillow, a toothbrush, toothpaste, floss, lip gloss, toiletries, a blow dryer, glasses or contact lens case, and so on.

- A camera, a video camera, a pad and a pencil, books, and magazines.

- A list of the phone numbers of family and friends.

- For the baby: an outfit, two receiving blankets, a hat, warm items if needed (such as sweaters, a heavy blanket, and so on), gentle baby wipes, Boppy (or another supportive breast-feeding pillow), and a baby book for footprints.

- For the car: two blankets, two towels (in case you are leaking breast milk), music.

Your Parting Words

Be sure to thank any and all people who assisted you in your labor. Remember that even if you didn't realize it, many people were concerned about you and your baby's care and well-being. Everyone was trying his or her best to ensure you a healthy labor. The people around you deserve acknowledgment for the contribution they made to your alignment and for being part of the realization of your context. You may not have seen them or been aware of them during labor, but I can assure you that your birth team and the facilities staff have put in a lot of hard work during your labor.

The skills you have learned in this process of alignment are crucial not only for childbirth; you will be able to use them to fulfill and create whatever you wish for the rest of your life, especially in developing lasting, strong relationships. Share these lessons with your children so that they can also learn to trust themselves and be able to communicate powerfully and clearly. This will help you create beautiful relationships with them, enabling them to be proud of themselves and manifest their dreams. We are all responsible for the lives we create. I hope these processes and ways of being will support you in everything that you do.

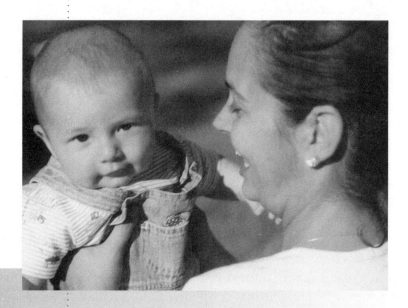

9 Getting Ready for Baby

Many people believe that once their baby is born, the hard work of pregnancy is over. Others decide, consciously or otherwise, to forgo preparing ahead of time for the first several months after the baby is born. But the thought of winging it may cause subconscious anxiety that you could take into childbirth. Just as you initially distinguished the context for your childbirth, it is now time to create a new context for the next phase of your life. This chapter focuses on the details you should consider now in order to create a context for after the birth. Just as you aligned with your birth team, you must align with a pediatrician. You will need to get your house in order and prepare yourself mentally and emotionally for the coming baby.

In essence, you need to create a plan, as best as you can in advance, for the first six weeks after the baby is born, as well as for the first year. It is so important for your peace of mind that you look at every area of your life in advance. Once you create a context for your new family, you need to be aligned with all of the details and the areas of life that you can make decisions about now. Then you will be ready to address any surprises that may come up, because the details and the "big picture" work have already been taken care of.

This new context will encompass goals you set for yourself as a parent, while you continue to incorporate the ideals of "family" into your life. Designing this particular context is a powerful exercise that can help you understand your visions about parenting and what kind of life you want to create for your child and yourself. So many people are unprepared for the future after their babies are born. The deep work on this context is necessary and is just a natural extension of everything you have done during pregnancy and childbirth.

As you think about your new family, decide what you want to create for everyone in it. Will your family be communicative, respectful, supporting, or protective? Will you be able to reach a level of deep understanding with your partner and your children? Do you want to have fun and spend time together, talk, and celebrate? Will you teach your children independence or show them the benefits of a strong sense of family? As you clarify what you want, your commitment will guide you through each choice for beginning your new family life.

You may also want to thinking about what kind of parent you want to be. For example, my context for being a parent is based on my commitment to guide and teach my children to trust themselves, know themselves, and make the best choices for themselves throughout their lives, which will make a big difference for others and for the world. The ways that I share this context with them include the actions I have taken from the beginning of their lives. My methods keep changing, but my commitment to this context remains the same.

There are so many cultural conversations about babies and parenting that *seem* true when you first hear them, but they are not by any means how every family has to look or act. I find each of the following statements to border on the negative, and I understand how they can infect your context. That's why it is so important to analyze each one and see whether it contains an underlying truth and whether it will apply to you. Look at the following statements, and see how you will shape your context in response to them:

- You will never sleep again.
- Your baby will always come first.
- Your marriage will deteriorate.
- There is never enough time.
- You won't have time to take care of yourself.
- Your body will never seem the same.
- Life is really going to change.

First, let's put each of these statements in perspective. Consider that every phase of your life is an important rite of passage that helps make up the story of your life. You are the author of your own story. So your life up to this point has been made up of a variety of chapters that tell that story. Having a baby is a new chapter. So each of these statements can be true, to some extent, but they don't have to be your perspective and experience about parenting or the truth about "what you will turn into." Imagine that each one can be taken as a point of reference for you to decide how important you will make it in your new context and how you will use it to create your own destiny. For example, your life is going to change. How can it be otherwise? But the questions you have to ask yourself are: Am I willing to change my life completely for this new baby, or will this baby find his or her way into my existing life? Or will the next phase of my life with a family have a whole new character?

My client Lia came up with the following text to clarify her parenting commitment to the baby boy she was going to birth. Her ideas can be used as a sample to help you get some clarity, taking it all one step at a time within your context and commitment:

- I am committed to learning my baby's signals so that I can teach him how to soothe himself. When it feels right, I will begin to teach him to sleep on a consistent schedule.

- I plan on taking care of myself by taking naps when the baby does in the first month so that I won't feel so tired.

- Our baby is important to us, but so is the foundation of our relationship and marriage. I will nurture my marriage by communicating regularly and honestly, and will make sure my husband and I take time for just the two of us, with at least one date night each week in the initial months after the birth.

- I will allow myself to find a new rhythm to balance all that is important to me—taking care of myself, my work, my relationship and friends. I realize that I may need support to do this.

- I am committed to breast-feeding.

- I will help bring my body into balance and recalibrate myself, eating healthy, nurturing foods.

- I will take the first six weeks to heal. Afterward, I will investigate exercise options. It might be yoga or fast walking with the baby in the stroller. I'm not sure yet but I am clear that exercise will be one of the ways that I will feel strong, and will help me feel good about the way I look.

- This is a new chapter in my life and I am excited about the adventures to come, the sweet new experiences, and growing in a way that will allow me to feel balanced and satisfied.

The New Family Plan

The new family plan affects everyone in your household, addressing the details you need to resolve after the childbirth and the decisions you must make. It focuses on the first six weeks after your baby arrives and includes issues surrounding the care of your infant as well as your life: your work, your lifestyle, your partner, and your new baby. Each of these issues will become part of your context for the first few months after your baby is born, and by addressing them, you will be able to relax once they are completed and have more time to bond with your new family.

The following template points toward some ideas for you to consider. This list enables you to determine the support you will need so that you can nurture yourself and become the best parent you can be. As you did with the birth plan, write out your responses to these prompts in the affirmative. This document is for you and your partner alone, but it will help you actually see the various aspects of your context.

- Are there children in your home? If so, are there special activities that they can engage in during this sensitive time for them?

- Are there members of your birth team or extended birth team who can take your children on special outings? Is there a special game or toy you can buy as a gift to give them immediately after the birth?

- Have you prepared the children for how to handle and interact with the new baby? Can you assign each of the siblings a simple job to do for the baby?

- Have you explained that you might initially be physically weaker and more tired than you usually are? Be clear with your children that you will be okay—there is no need for them to worry.

- Who will be cooking the meals? Can you ask someone on your birth team to arrange for a food chain, in which friends, family members, or neighbors bring over big lunches or dinners for the first few weeks? During your third trimester, have this person create a schedule for meals so that after you give birth, the schedule is in place. There are also great resources, such as Peapod, that deliver grocery items and healthy, nutritious foods. (See the Resources section at the end of the book.)

- Who will run errands for you?

- Can members of your birth team come to visit or give you a short break at least three to four times a week, so that you can take a bath or a nap or grab a movie with your partner?

- Would you like to hire a postpartum doula or baby nurse? Arrange to make phone interviews a few weeks before your due date, or even earlier, so that if you need one, you can make this decision effortlessly.

- Can your partner take a few days off work immediately after the birth? A week? Some companies do have paternity leave for husbands.

- Will you be breast-feeding? Do you have the number for the La Leche League hotline in your area? (See the Resources section in the back of the book.) Do you have phone numbers of lactation consultants whom you could call for advice or to schedule a home visit? As with the postpartum doula, it is possible for you to have quick phone conversations with two to three lactation consultants before your due date so that if you need such help, you can easily reach out to someone you trust.

- Do you have pets that will need care or walking? Can someone in your neighborhood or a professional dog walker do this for you during the first six weeks after the baby's birth?

- Have you chosen a pediatrician? (See page 238 for more details.)

- Are you interested in herbal remedies to help your healing after birth? Will you need to order these products online or is there a health food store in your area? (See the Resources section in the back of this book.)

- Where will the new baby sleep? Do you wish to have your new child sleep with you in your bed or in a crib next to the bed? If there are any siblings, inform them of your intentions about the new sleeping arrangements beforehand.

- Do you wish to have visitors? Or would you rather have minimal interactions with others until everyone in your new family has gotten better acquainted with one another? Are you not sure? Discuss this with friends and family so that they are sensitive to this special time in your life.

- If you do want to have visitors, are there certain rules you would like them to follow, such as washing their hands before touching the baby, helping themselves to food and drink in your home so that you don't have to bother with serving them, and making an effort to speak and play with your other children, if you have any?

- Who will do the laundry? Is there a laundry service in your neighborhood that you can rely on for pick-up and drop-off?
- If you need a babysitter, have you found one you can trust?
- Have you researched the child-care and daycare options in your area?
- Would you and your partner like to go on a date? Or merely spend a quiet night at home with each other? Maybe you would like to eat at a nice restaurant or see a movie, a concert, or a performance?
- Will you be exercising or stretching and when?
- Are you interested in staying connected to the outside world? Do you want friends from work to tell you about what is going on there?
- What baby-related activities do you need to learn more about or see demonstrations of? These may include the proper bathing of the baby, taking the baby's temperature, breast-feeding techniques, formula-feeding techniques, the care of the infant's nails, developmental and health milestones, umbilical cord care, circumcision care, calming a fretful baby, and diapering.

Postpartum Doulas

A postpartum doula offers emotional and physical comfort and informational support to families at home after the baby is born. Many doulas are both birth and postpartum doulas, but the majority chooses one role or the other.

DONA International, the oldest, largest, and most respected doula association in the world, suggests that postpartum doulas do whatever a family needs to best enjoy and care for the new baby. This can include sharing information about baby care, as well as assisting with breast-feeding education and making sure that the mother is fed, well hydrated, and comfortable. Unlike a baby nurse, a postpartum doula focuses on the mother as well as on the baby.

A postpartum doula can stay with a family anywhere from one or two visits to more than three months. Some of them work full days; others work three- to five-hour shifts during the day or the evenings; and some work overnight.

If you can't afford a postpartum doula or simply don't want one, you can also count on the women in your tribe. One of my close girlfriends helped me so much during the first week with my baby. This is such an important time for you to ask for the support you need and to connect with your friends and family; it can make all the difference. Remember the members of your tribe, and call on them when you need them. Don't be afraid to ask for help. Your tribe should include women who will mother you once the baby arrives. Some of these women should be mothers themselves, because they will understand exactly what you are going through and will honor your wishes and needs. They will make sure you've eaten, had a shower, gotten some fresh air, and have company so that you're not alone and overwhelmed. Find out who will be available and when, so that when you need someone, she can come right away.

Meet Sally

While planning a home birth, Sally hadn't thought that she'd need a postpartum doula. She and her partner were focusing solely on the birth and were firmly grounded in their choice of a midwife and a labor doula. But since Sally's mother had not breast-fed her children, she wanted to have someone guide and coach her daughter after the birth of her first grandchild. She gave Sally a gift of several sessions of postpartum mentoring and breast-feeding support.

Sally hired Ina Bransome for the job. Ina laid out her vision of what would happen after the birth. She explained that she would help the new parents enjoy the first weeks of living together with their child. Her first two visits encouraged Sally to simply be with her son: forget about a normal sense of time and turn the clock faces to the wall (as they did during the labor and the birth), so that Sally could join this new person in the eternal present he was living in. Following the baby's lead, Ina had Sally sleep intermittently, rest with him, and live at his pace. Ina helped with the learning curve of breast-feeding, while giving Sally gentle assistance. She also taught Sally and her partner some of her own techniques for creating soothing sounds to help trigger the calming reflex; how to hit the pause button in a crying jag; ways to hold the baby that would give him a long-lasting sense of security and closeness; how to make sounds to signal when you are offering the baby a change in position or activity; and encouragement to Dad and Mom as they increasingly gained skill and confidence in their parenting. Ina taught them the signs that newborns use to show that they're satisfied, when they are experiencing pleasure, or when they're becoming uncomfortable.

As an experienced "poopologist," Ina helped the parents track the shift from colostrum to mature breast milk by reading the baby's increasingly yellow stool. Ina loaned them a sling from her daughter Haya's vast inventory so that from the first days, they could tote their son along with them as they resumed walking through the neighborhood. In later sessions during the first week, Ina helped Sally give the baby his first sponge bath and monitored the umbilical cord healing. Sally believes that it was invaluable having someone so knowledgeable to talk with, because there were so many decisions she had to make. Having a highly experienced postpartum doula such as Ina check in with the family and monitor everyone's progress, sharing tips and a greater depth of understanding, was a huge relief during the first few weeks of the baby's life.

Choosing a Pediatrician

Now is the time to research, interview, and choose a pediatrician for your child. You want to make this decision in your final months of pregnancy, so that your pediatrician will be able to see the baby either in the hospital or after your home birth. The first place to start is by asking your trusted, like-minded friends for referrals. If you are moving or new to a town, you can ask the hospital or the birthing center for a list of pediatricians who are affiliated with it, regardless of whether you will be birthing at that location. Choose a pediatrician who is local to you. Check his or her policies on after-hours phone calls, weekend appointments, and office procedures.

Although it is nice for you to enjoy being with your pediatrician, it is more important that you see whether you can trust this person and his or her decision-making skills. The main thing you will want to decide is whether your pediatrician resonates with your current context and parenting philosophy. Ask potential pediatricians, for example, whether they have children of their own, and what their philosophy is regarding child rearing. Find out whether they encourage new mothers to breast-feed and for how long. See whether you can garner details about their lives, such as their opinions on scheduled naps and feedings, co-sleeping arrangements (where the child sleeps in the same bed with his or her parents), and their recommendations for babies who cry when they're put to sleep at night. Make sure to address medical issues as well, including each doctor's beliefs about antibiotics, vaccinations, and circumcision.

You are entitled to know the doctors' current rates, what types of insurance they take, and the average length of time they allocate for sick and well visits. You should also find out whether they share a practice, and if so, how sick visits are handled. (In other words, will you always see the same doctor?)

I love my pediatrician, Dr. Michel Cohen, who is the author of a book called *The New Basics: A–Z Baby & Child Care for the Modern Parent*. His thinking, philosophy, spirit, and personality have worked well for me and my family. He and his team are always accessible and respond quickly when I have a question or a concern. He believes that most childhood illnesses are simple and self-resolving. Parents should be vigilant in monitoring symptoms but should also respect the body's natural defenses and avoid unnecessary or even detrimental interventions. This resonates completely with my context for raising my children.

Nesting

Around the fifth month of pregnancy, your nesting instinct may begin to take hold. Nesting refers to an uncontrollable urge to clean house, tie up the loose ends of old projects, and organize your world in preparation for the new baby. Interestingly, many females in the animal kingdom have this same innate need. Just as you see birds making their nests, mothers-to-be do exactly the same thing. During this time, you may feel the need to gather up the equipment you will want for your baby. Or, you may want to retreat into the comforts of home and familiar company, like a brooding hen. This can be very relaxing and comforting. When it occurs around forty weeks into pregnancy, the nesting urge can also signal the onset of labor.

The act of nesting puts you in control of your environment and provides a sense of accomplishment as you progress toward child-birth. It can be really funny to watch some women nesting: they might spend hours perfecting every corner of their homes or may focus on creating impeccable pantries (as if it never mattered so much before). I've heard women say that they feel as if they are under a spell in which they feel unstoppable.

It can also be therapeutic to intensely prepare for your baby. Carl Jung, the famous Swiss psychiatrist, had his own ritual, which I've adopted. When he was trying to work through an emotional problem or felt upset about something that he could not get clear about, he engaged in physical activity. He found that when he did something physical, the answers and the clarity he was looking for came to him.

I refer to this practice metaphorically as "playing in the sandbox." Nesting is a form of "playing in the sandbox" because it lets you focus on the physical, thereby creating an empty mental space to allow for ideas, solutions, and answers to arise. Nesting then becomes a tool that is consistent with everything you do and create in using this book.

Nesting is another dimension of the bond you make with your baby. You are preparing yourself physically as well emotionally in these final stages of your pregnancy, as you deeply relax and focus on your future. For many women, this level of preparation lets them envision what their lives will look like. Pregnancy can at times be very amorphous: you know the baby is coming, but you can't quite wrap your mind around it because you can't see it. Think of nesting as creating a special welcome for the baby. It is a perfect way to become prepared and to connect with yourself, your baby, the flow of your new lifestyle, and the divinity of motherhood.

What You Need to Buy

Babies really don't take up much space, but their equipment sure does! Here are the most important pieces of baby equipment that you'll need. There are many resources for all of these items at the end of this book, including Ali Wing's great book *Giggle Guide to Baby Gear.* Ali is the founder and CEO of Giggle Stores.

- A rear-facing car seat that meets current safety guidelines (not the one your cousin bought ten years ago and is bequeathing to you)
- A crib
- A breast pump and storage bags for breast milk if you plan to breast-feed
- Bottles
- Infant formula if you will not breast-feed
- A stroller
- A chair that you can comfortably sit in while you feed the baby
- A sling or some form of a baby carrier
- A baby monitor (if you live in a large, expansive home)
- A high chair (for later, when the baby can sit up by herself)
- A fully stocked diaper bag (I recommend two if you have a car—it's always great to have a backup)
- Diapers, wipes, and diaper rash ointment
- Infant nail scissors
- Seasonally appropriate clothes
- Baby blankets
- Burping cloths
- Towels specifically for the baby
- A baby hair brush
- A rocker for the baby
- SafetyMate for the new parent: Talking first aid (available at www.safetymate.com)

Here are some additional items that are purely optional:

- A baby basket/Moses basket/bassinet
- A changing table
- A baby swing
- Pacifiers
- A food processor/blender or food grinder to make your own baby food
- Toys—a rattle, a mobile, books, visual-stimulation toys
- Music for the baby's room and for you

Your Life during the First Month

Mothering is more instinctual and emotional than anything you may have been required to do in the workplace. Communicating with your infant for the first few weeks is more physical and emotional than verbal. At the same time, you may not feel like talking to others. When I had my first child, I was surprised to find that I didn't want to talk with a lot of people or return calls, because normally I am a very verbal person. I took that first month to be quieter and connect with the baby and my new family. I felt highly emotional, deeply sensitive, and intuitive, which were all normal and common responses. My intuition was a gift, and I wanted to bathe in it, use it, and appreciate it, as well as protect it.

Even though I had tried to prepare for what my life would be like, I was still surprised by the day-to-day aspects. I remember that my favorite quote from that time came from the writer Anne Lamott. In her classic book on infancy, *Operating Instructions*, she wrote, "I just can't get over how much babies cry. I really had no idea what I was getting into. To tell you the truth, I thought it would be more like getting a cat."

Newborns sleep fewer than two hours at a time, so you will probably experience some sleep deprivation. Combined with your fluctuating hormone levels, this will take a toll on your ability to think rationally. Remember that this mental fog is normal and part of the journey, so please give yourself some credit and keep this in perspective. You are hard at work learning about your baby and figuring out a whole new language of behavior. Take to heart the fact that with time, your faster, more logical way of processing and verbalizing will return. Finally, a lack of sleep might make you irritable at times, so if you snap, apologize right away or see whether you can catch yourself beforehand. My motto is "Never ruin an apology with an excuse." If you see that you are in a foul mood, spend extra time taking care of yourself, so that you can be a better mother and enjoy your family.

Set up your life so that at least for the first month, you can be at ease with this experience and flow with it. I really think that nature has designed you and this process to be like this. For example, try to sleep when the baby sleeps. Don't expect to get a lot done during this time, except eating, sleeping, and being with your family. Everything else can wait. Your sheets certainly don't have to be ironed. Follow the advice of the Buddha: "Eat when you're hungry. Drink when you're thirsty. Sleep when you're tired."

You want to create a rhythm for the baby's eating and sleeping schedules over the first few weeks. Again, you will be learning your baby's temperament, communication, and signals, which will help you create a balance between offering the baby comfort and figuring out limits. You will come to know how your baby likes to be held during feeding, how long the feeding lasts, and when and how she needs to be burped. Babies vary in their eating schedules, but once you discover your baby's rhythm, you will be able to trust your instincts.

There are many schools of thought when it comes to establishing sleeping schedules. These range from attachment parenting (where you sleep with your child) to the Ferber technique (letting your baby cry until he can learn to soothe himself). These are all personal decisions you need to make. There are very specific instructions for "sleep training" in a few books I love, such as *A Mother's Circle* by Soho Parenting Center and *The Secret of the Baby Whisperer* by Tracy Hogg.

I breast-fed my first child and brought her into bed with me, which I found to be very convenient and beautiful. She slept with me for months. But as great as this felt, it was a very difficult habit to break. She came to rely on me in order to fall asleep, and she used me to soothe herself. About a year later, she was still sleeping in my bed, and I realized that I had to teach her to fall asleep on her own. This was so, so hard for me. After I fed her in a beautiful chair in her room and placed her in her cozy crib, I then had to endure listening to her cry. So when my second child arrived, I still breast-fed him and was very connected to him, but I made sure that he felt nurtured right in his own bed from the start.

Babies thrive on regular routines and learn to anticipate them. Your baby will recognize a nightly routine as a signal that it is time to go to bed. I always started the routine with an evening bath. You can design your own from here: soft cozy clothes, music, ambiance, gentle rocking, massaging, and an extra dose of physical touch before the child is willing to let go for the night. My friend Marcia Norman, who was part of my tribe, taught me about her bedtime ritual with her kids. She called it a "tickle back"—it is a very light touch massage with the tips of your fingers on your baby's back: so relaxing and soothing. My kids still ask for their tickle backs at bedtime today.

The Blend Theory

One of the best pieces of advice I can pass on to you is from a great friend and tribe member, Pam Wolf. She is the owner of the New York Kids Club and a mother of four children. She taught me the "blend" theory, which she invented and I love. The blend theory is when people blend their time together for various things/activities/elements of their lives, hoping that if they throw everything together, something good will come out of it. Usually, that doesn't happen, and everyone feels as if he or she has been done a disservice and you feel as if you are going crazy. Her advice is to run the other way: make clear choices when you have to divide your time so that you don't blend things together. For example, when you are feeding the baby, do only that: don't try and have an important conversation with your husband, feed the cat, or take a phone call. When you are going on a date with your husband, really be with him and enjoy your time together.

Working against the blend theory allows you to create time for each of the things you love. It will really make you reevaluate what is profoundly important to you and will give you the opportunity to let go of what is not essential. I use this way of thinking even now. When my kids come home from school, I spend time with them. I don't try to check my e-mail or talk on the phone at the same time. Instead, I'm really with them, and they feel this and appreciate my undivided attention. The same goes for my work: when I am with clients or writing, I am working and my family knows not to interrupt me unless it is an emergency. This kind of single-minded focus allows you to be efficient and truly in the moment. Best of all, you can include the blend theory in your life now as you prepare for your childbirth.

The Gift of Prioritizing

Your pregnancy is such a great opportunity to reevaluate and assess every aspect of your life. Some of my clients have used this time to reexamine their careers and the value and satisfaction they derive from their jobs. Others choose not to return to work, some return to work in a modified way, and a few continue to work full time. See what works best for you and your lifestyle.

As you consider your priorities, remember that one of the most important responsibilities of your new life is to mother yourself and create balance. Look to those you love and admire as role models. See how they balance family, work, and meeting their own needs. Then turn the mirror toward yourself to reflect the light of those same ideas. It can be quite a revelation to see yourself in this nourishing light.

Achieving balance encompasses all of the emotional, mental, and physical work you have been doing throughout your pregnancy. Every aspect of your being will change yet again once the baby arrives. Physically, your body will dramatically transform as you shed your pregnancy weight. Be patient with yourself, yet at the same time do what is necessary to make yourself feel good. Take care of yourself and eat highly nutritious meals, especially if you are nursing. You can begin an exercise program after the first six weeks. Exercise of any sort will give you increased energy, restored muscle tone, and a renewed sense of confidence in your body and yourself. There are many good ways to get back into shape like taking power walks with your baby in the stroller, yoga classes, and more.

It is not true that you cannot get back into great shape after pregnancy. I honestly got into the best shape of my life after giving birth. There are many great classes and experts devoted to helping women get back into shape after pregnancy, including Brett Hoebel of Hoebel Fitness in New York City. He helps his clients, which include Veronica Webb, the model, journalist, and television personality, transform their postpartum bodies into their best bodies ever. To do so, he deals with the mental, emotional, and physical contexts of his clients. Women can be frustrated that they gained weight and are weaker than before their pregnancy, but Brett gives them perspective. His message is to be patient and kind to yourself. Remember, it took nine months to put weight on, and losing a pound per week is average and safe. Hormonal imbalances as well as anxiety can impact weight-loss progress. Brett's exercise regimen focuses on strengthening the core, and strength training with slower movements for the four to six weeks after delivery.

Many studies have shown that women are more physically resilient after having children—some of the best woman marathoners are those who already have children. You can write your own visualizations to focus on how you'll want to look and the sense of vitality you'll want to feel within yourself, as well as with your partner and your children. Be gentle in the beginning and know that you can create the body, the vitality, and the good health you desire. Breast-feeding will not only enable you to shed your pregnancy weight, it also helps you balance your emotions. While you are nursing, you will continue to produce high levels of oxytocin, "the happy hormone." This will relax you and keep you calm. Strive to overcome self-critical feelings. You are taking on so much right now: caring for your baby, providing warmth and security. More than anyone else ever can, the baby needs you. She loves and appreciates you, and you should love yourself as well.

Balance also means that you need to think of yourself sometimes. New mothers are often so busy taking care of their babies that they don't take time for themselves. This includes nurturing your relationship with your partner. Your partnership should evolve with your new life. It is important to carve out a part of each day that is a special time for you and your partner. Creating structure and schedules for the baby will also give you more freedom: once you establish a rhythm for your baby's feeding and sleeping schedules, there will be a block of time in the evening that you can reclaim as yours. You and your partner will need to work as a team in raising this child. Clear, open, respectful communication is crucial for everyone to know what he or she is doing for the team. You need to align on every aspect and decide who does what best, then make that person accountable for those duties. If you and your partner can look at all of the necessary tasks—paying bills, middle-of-the-night feedings, grocery shopping, washing the dishes—you can divide these chores equitably so that no one feels put upon. You both may feel intense emotions about how you are doing as parents, and you may dwell on this issue. Be gentle with yourselves and with each other—parenting is a learned art that does not always come naturally to either sex. Through your respect, communication, and compassion, you will be able to talk through aligning your parenting styles, based on the context you created for yourselves as parents and the context for your family.

The Language of Love

Connecting with, loving, and teaching your baby will be an amazing journey. Your baby's rapid physical development during the first year forms the basis for the unfolding of the child's intelligence in the years that follow. In addition, your baby is beginning to develop emotionally and socially, and the lessons about love and trust that are learned as an infant form a foundation for later emotional health. There is no doubt that infants thrive on love. Countless studies have shown that love, touch, and care are vital. Show care and affection to your baby throughout the day. Sing, chat, and play as you get to know each other. Leave the infant in peace and quiet to sleep or, when she is awake, let her get to know herself in calm surroundings without constant distractions. Often, it is very difficult to show the infant this respect and leave her alone. If you must keep satisfying your own need for reassurance by looking at and interacting with your beautiful baby, this might hinder the infant's ability to be contented within herself. Trust yourself and the baby will trust.

The love and the bond that you will feel are indescribable and unique to you and your baby. So much will unfold, and all of it is accompanied by love as you discover your baby's spirit and personality while she sleeps, feeds, and holds you, with her tiny hand gripping yours. Make sure you are in a place of love as you burp the baby, change diapers, oversee baths, watch her discover shapes, and wipe her tush over and over again—now, that is love. The baby will respond to you with love as she begins to smile, laugh, teethe, enjoy music, handle toys, become physically stronger and more agile, discover foods, and maybe even walk. Loving interaction is a crucial component of the baby's development, sense of ease, peacefulness, and self-awareness.

Enjoy all of it and be present to it; each phase is precious. Many people say that it goes so fast—it does, if you are not present. So the key to feeling joy in your baby's first year is for you to be present—live in the moment and keep a sense of humor.

Feeding Yourself

When your new baby arrives, the last thing you want to do is cook. And yet you need to stay nourished. Karen Gurwitz, the author of *The Well-Rounded Pregnancy Cookbook*, prepared this short list of things you can do to pull together quick and easy meals:

- Keep canned beans on hand for a quick meal of beans and rice. Smaller legumes, such as lentils and adzuki beans, are good choices because they minimize bloating.

- Keep dried fruit available for a fiber-rich snack that will satisfy your sweet tooth. You can also try Xocai, a delicious extremely dark chocolate that is manufactured without processed sugar. It is high in anti-oxidants, which energize the body's immune system.

- Oatmeal is high in fiber and makes a nourishing breakfast.

- Another one of my favorite recipes for breakfast is made by scrambling eggs (two eggs or just the egg whites of two eggs) with dried oatmeal. Add a touch of lecithin, a tablespoon or more of ground flaxseeds, some maca (a super food), and a drop of flaxseed oil in the pan and stir it all up creating a healthy "pancake." Kids love it too.

- Whole grains such as brown rice, quinoa, and whole-wheat pasta can be topped off with your favorite jar of tomato sauce for a quick lunch.

- Keeping yourself well-hydrated is crucial, especially if you are breast-feeding. Eat plenty of greens and grains, which will help you produce milk.

- Stock your freezer so that you have all of the foods that you really rely on. Precut and prewash vegetables, then dry and freeze them for later use. Frozen, store-bought vegetables are absolutely fine. If I had to name one vegetable that every woman should incorporate into her diet when she is pregnant and nursing, it would be kale. It is so powerful in terms of nutrients that it really makes a big difference.

- When people ask what they can bring for you or the baby, ask for green salads.

Things I Wish I Had Known Then

- Give Boirum Chamomile liquid capsules to the baby to help with teething—these were lifesavers for me. They are homeopathic, are made of pure chamomile, and ease the pain of teething.

- Learn to swaddle your baby—it is so comforting for him.

- Use a baby carrier when you want to soothe the baby and do things around the house; it allows him to get the comforting he needs and leaves your hands free for everything else.

- Take a nap every afternoon, at least during the first month. Give Dad a turn at napping as well.

- Don't make promises you can't keep. Know and accept your limitations.

- Prioritize.

- Ask for help. Call on your tribe when life gets overwhelming.

- Spend time with your partner and good friends. Don't center every minute of your life around your newborn.

- Pamper yourself. Get a massage, a manicure, a facial, a pedicure, or get your hair done. Whatever makes you feel special, cared for, and beautiful—do it!

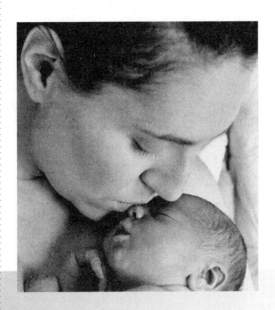

10 *Surrender* Means Letting Go

Now that you are fully educated about what can happen to your mind and body during delivery, it's time to revisit your context. Take this opportunity to create a final mental checklist, and make sure that there are no issues left unanswered or unaligned. By the end of this chapter, you will be able to declare yourself complete, meaning that you have done all of the physical as well as the mental work necessary to prepare for the arrival of your child. All of this work will allow you to fully let go when you give birth.

Your Final Checklist

Use the following checklist to ensure you have addressed every aspect of this childbirth. Do a mental inventory and make sure you have everything you need to be confident and prepared. As you look at where you are right now, remember not to judge or invalidate yourself: you have made many difficult decisions, and you should be proud of all of them. Let yourself appreciate everything you have already done and created. At the same time, keep your mind open to adjust or recalibrate what you need or want from this point forward.

Use the following list and rate each category on a scale of 1 to 10: "10" means that you feel completely at peace with the issue and know that you have done all you need and want to do in this area. You feel empowered, free, and proud of yourself. On the other hand, a "1" would signify that you have barely touched this issue at all. Next, try to determine exactly what it would take to bring each area up to a "10." What will you need to do in the next few weeks to be complete? Then, create a plan for each area. Write down your intentions, and devise a way to ensure that every area listed here becomes a "10."

1. *Creating the context for your birth.* You should be clear about your context and how to fulfill it. You'll need to fully tease it out, which includes distinguishing all of the words you used to describe it. You should also be in alignment with your partner and your birth team about your context. You should be able to communicate it clearly and know that you have been heard. You can feel, see, and know every aspect of this context. If you are not at a 9 or a 10 at this point, use the toolbox again. Try some of the art exercises, such as making a collage, so that you can convey a vision of your context. Continue to work with your partner and practice the art of communication, as discussed in chapter 8, so that you feel more confident that your voice will be heard when you express your intentions for this birth.

2. *Aligning your birth team.* Your birth plan should be complete. You should have a document that clearly outlines all of your wishes for this birth. Make sure you have addressed everything you need to feel safe and confident. Is there anything left that you are not dealing with, feel uncomfortable with, skipped over, assumed, have a bad feeling about, or are not sure of? Now is the time to be completely honest with yourself. Remember that you can deal with almost everything in life by

communicating clearly, so it is vital that you use this deep level of honesty with yourself, your partner, and your birth team. If there is more to ask or talk about, make a final list of all the conversations you need to have, no matter how simple the topics are. These conversations may be with your extended birth team, such as family members and friends who will be around you afterward. The courage that it takes to have these conversations will require you to tap into your well of confidence.

3. *Review your plans for when the baby arrives.* Revisit the checklist in chapter 9 that covers the first six weeks after the baby is born. Make sure you fully understand why each of these decisions is important and what they will look like. If there are still decisions that remain to be made, continue to research your options until you feel that they are complete and finalized.

4. *Review your weekly practice using the toolbox.* Can you tell which exercises are working for you, enabling you to relax? Which ones should you focus on now and which ones for the childbirth? First, determine what you need to focus on right now. I recommend that you exponentially increase the practices that you love to do in months 7, 8, and 9. For example, if you are meditating or using visualizations about two or three times a week, increase this to once a day in months 8 and 9, even if you spend only a few minutes on it each time. Make sure that you continue to incorporate some physical activity into your daily practice. Most of all, continue to take care of yourself. If you have enjoyed prenatal massages, get a few more of them in month 8 and even more in month 9. Allow yourself to enjoy and bask in the last month of your pregnancy, as you learn to honor yourself and your baby.

5. *Reconsider any remaining personal issues.* Do you still have unresolved fears, concerns, or negative thoughts regarding this birth or your life after the baby appears? If so, I recommend that you go back to chapter 1 and work with the fear-releasing exercises. See whether you notice anything different when you do these exercises again. Do the same thoughts, feelings,

or images come up for you, or have you uncovered new issues that you need to address? I know that when I do these exercises, if I come up with the same thoughts, complaints, or fears more than a few times, this is a signal to me that I have to do something about them. Most often, I need to have a conversation with someone or take a certain action. So if you notice this pattern with yourself, don't procrastinate. Take care of yourself and your needs now.

How Did Your Own Birth Go?

If you have never heard your own birth story, now is a great time to uncover it. Ask your mother how you were born and what it was like for her. There is no guarantee that you will give birth the way your mother did, but you may discover unconscious suggestions and connections.

Many of my clients have been so emotionally connected to their mothers that they were unconsciously attempting to bring these relationships into their personal birthing and parenting experiences. For example, Martine once realized during a meditation that she was thinking about the fact that her mom gave birth to her by Cesarean. Her mother had passed away about a year prior to the meditation, and they had been very close. Martine discovered that subconsciously, she was planning to have a C-section as a way to connect with and honor her mother. Understanding this connection was important for Martine, and I helped her recognize that her child's birth will be distinct from her love for her mother. I showed her that for all of us, our past need not dictate our future.

Learn to Let Go

The final piece in the BornClear program is learning to let go. In preparing yourself for childbirth and parenting, you have gone through a series of stages as you worked through this book: first, you were able to get clear on your context; then you learned how to empower yourself through education, achieving clarity; and finally you were able to trust yourself and your choices. Once you have achieved this deep level of trust, you are now ready to surrender to the birth.

Letting go is perhaps one of the most difficult challenges you face. It is human nature to become easily and all too eagerly attached to things, people, and expectations. When you realize the inner power you possess, you can let go of your attachments. This doesn't mean that you don't work your hardest for the highest outcome, but rather that you do your best and leave the rest to whatever you define as divinity and what is meant to be.

You can be completely committed to your context and plan for your birth to go a certain way. The trick is not to become too attached to believing that this is the only way it should go or should look. That's the key about letting go. You can't predict the future, and every birth is different, so you can only do your best to prepare for what is to come. At the moment that you go into labor, you will need to let go of your expectations and accept the birth, knowing that you did everything you could to make it the best possible experience it could be. All the work you have done so far, your thinking, reading, being conscious, bonding with your baby, taking care of yourself, and relaxing, has already helped you to become a loving and conscious parent. You have nurtured this little person for the last nine months, and all the while you have been reinventing a new paradigm for parenting, setting the tone for your baby's life. The birth is just one aspect of this journey; another is the life you are fashioning through the tone of your pregnancy, for yourself, your family, and your baby.

Resisting, holding on, controlling, feeling dependent, and being attached are the opposite of letting go. Letting go does not mean giving up or showing weakness, apathy, indifference, or carelessness. Instead, it reveals your deepest faith and trust in yourself. Be willing to let go of the childbirth you have planned and allow the childbirth that will be. As Joseph Campbell said, "We must be willing to let go of the life we have planned, so as to accept the life that is waiting for us."

If you cultivate this inner virtue of surrendering, you will become more patient, tolerant, empathetic, accepting, and open-minded in every aspect of your life, beginning with your childbirth. So with this final bit of preparation, give up any final resistance and let be what will be. As you "master" letting go, remember to acknowledge yourself up to this point of your journey. Acknowledge the parent you've already become and the consciousness that you have brought to this role. Be proud of yourself, no matter what the outcome of the actual birth is.

Once you are wholeheartedly able to surrender, know that you are fully prepared for birth. You are now complete and ready. Experience your gratitude for the journey, the lessons, and the love.

Meet Angelica

When I worked with Angelica on creating the context for her birth, she knew that she wanted it to be a very calm, Zenlike birth. One of her greatest concerns was that she was a control freak (as we all can be)—she called herself this and felt that she would have to deal with this controlling aspect of her personality and overcome it. She knew that this behavior affected every area of her life.

I told Angelica that she had to learn to surrender. This would be difficult for her: even when she went to prenatal yoga classes, there was this picture of a surrender motif and she could never really get it. Over the course of her sessions, I was able to explain to Angelica what surrendering truly looked and felt like. So when she went into labor, her practice of surrendering set the tone for her entire birth.

Later, Angelica told me that surrendering is what her childbirth taught her. She viewed it as the gift she gave herself, and she continued to use this new power and knowledge as she mothered her newborn baby, Ruby Elaine. She said, "When labor began, I was completely conscious of how the concept of surrender manifested itself. Perhaps it was like viewing a map of something but then actually being there and learning your way around. It was the key to allowing labor to unfold in the most meaningful way. I was able to fully conceptualize what surrender meant by going through the birth process. Before that, I had been able to envision it in some respects and apply it in certain situations throughout pregnancy, but until the point of my labor, surrender was not fully realized in terms of its potential as a labor tool and then later as a motif for life and mothering. As the journey of motherhood has unfolded, surrender as a recurring theme has been key to the experience. It has made itself apparent in its applicability to every aspect of my life: interpersonal relationships, public interactions (taking buses, waiting in bank lines, and so on), marriage . . . and the list goes on."

For Angelica, the lessons of surrender have shed a new light and given her a new perspective on how she views herself, her life, and people and how she mothers her child at every stage of their lives.

BornClear Is a Better Birth

By committing to this program, you have taken a major step toward developing yourself as a responsible and interactive being in this world. You have also begun a journey in conscious parenting. You have taken your fate into your own hands and squared it firmly with your beliefs. You have sparked a wheel of light that will pass through to your child for him or her to hold on to forever. Each being who follows in your line will carry the beauty of your personal power, one that you honed and mastered through the divinity of childbirth. Nothing will ever reverse this accomplishment. You have made a solid contribution to better the world by delivering to it a child who has been born clear.

Congratulations, and thank you!

Resources

Midwives

Foundation for the Advancement of Midwifery (FAM)
877-594-9996
http://www.formidwifery.org/

American College of Nurse-Midwives (ACNM)
240-485-1800
http://www.acnm.org/

Citizens for Midwifery (CfM)
888-CfM-4880 (236-4880)
http://www.cfmidwifery.org/

Midwives Alliance of North America (MANA)
888-923-MANA (6262)
http://www.mana.org/

National Association of Certified Professional Midwives (NACPM)
866-704-9844
http://www.nacpm.org/

The Farm
http://www.thefarm.org/

Advocacy

The Birth Survey
http://www.thebirthsurvey.com/

Childbirth Connection
212-777-5000
http://www.childbirthconnection.org/

The Coalition for Improving Maternity Services (CIMS)
888-282-CIMS (2467)
http://www.motherfriendly.org/

Choices in Childbirth (CIC)
212-983-4122
http://www.choicesinchildbirth.org/

National Advocates for Pregnant Women (NAPW)
212-255-9252
http://www.advocatesforpregnantwomen.org/

BirthNetwork
888-452-4784
http://www.birthnetwork.org/

Maternity Center Association
212-777-5000
http://www.maternitywise.org/

International Cesarean Awareness Network (ICAN)
800-686-ICAN
http://www.ican-online.org/

National Organization of
Circumcision Information Resource
Center (NOCIRC)
415-488-9883
nocirc@concentric.net
http://www.nocirc.org/

World Health Organization (WHO)
(+ 41 22) 791 21 11
http://www.who.int/en/

American College of Obstetricians
and Gynecologists (ACOG)
202-638-5577
http://www.acog.org/

Primal Health Resource Center
Dr. Michel Odent
http://www.birthworks.org/

National Organization of Mothers
of Twins Clubs, Inc. (NOMTC)
Executive Office
248-231-4480
http://www.nomotc.org/

MomsRising
http://www.momsrising.org/

International Center for Traditional
Childbirth (ICTC)
503-460-9324
http://www.blackmidwives.org/

National Women's Health
Information Center
800-994-9662
http://www.4Women.gov/

National Latina Institute for
Reproductive Health
212-422-2553
http://www.latinainstitute.org/

SisterSong: Women of Color
Reproductive Health Collective
404-756-2680
http://www.sistersong.net/

Family and Parenting Coaching

Bambini Consulting
Cinzia Fisher
619-723-0110
http://www.bambiniconsulting.com/

Family Voices, Inc.
888-835-5669
http://www.familyvoices.org/

Gay Parent Magazine
718-380-1780
http://www.gayparentmag.com/

Alternative Medicine Organizations

American Association of
Naturopathic Physicians (AANP)
202-237-8150 or 866-538-2267
http://www.naturopathic.org/

American Botanical Council (ABC)
512-926-4900
http://abc.herbalgram.org/

American Herbalists Guild
203-272-6731
http://www.americanherbalist.com/

American Holistic Medical
Association (AHMA)
440-838-1010
http://www.holisticmedicine.org/

The American Institute of
Homeopathy (AIH)
888-445-9988
http://www.homeopathyusa.org/

Association for Prenatal & Perinatal
Psychology & Health (APPPH)
707-887-2838
http://www.birthpsychology.com/

The Biodynamic Craniosacral
Therapy Association of North
America (BCTA/NA)
734-904-0546
http://www.craniosacraltherapy.org/

International Chiropractic Pediatric
Association (ICPA)
610-565-2360
http://www.icpa4kids.com/

North American Society of
Homeopaths (NASH)
206-720-7000
http://www.homeopathy.org/

Holistic Moms Network (HMN)
877-HOL-MOMS (465-6667)
http://www.holisticmoms.org/

Holistic Pediatric Association (HPA)
707-237-5312
http://www.hpakids.com/

International Federation of
Aromatherapists (IMA)
(+44 20) 8992 9605
http://www.ifaroma.org/

National Association for Holistic
Aromatherapy (NAHA)
509-325-3419
http://www.naha.org/

National Certification Commission
for Acupuncture and Oriental
Medicine (NCCAOM)
904-598-1005
http://www.nccaom.org/

Birth Center Resources

American Association of Birth
Centers (AABC)
215-234-8068
http://www.birthcenters.org/

Breast-Feeding Support

The Academy of Breastfeeding
Medicine (ABM)
800-990-4ABM (4226) (toll free)
800-994-9662 (multilingual info line)
http://www.bfmed.org/

Adoptive Breastfeeding Resource
Website
http://www.fourfriends.com/abrw/

Breastfeeding.com
720-304-3112
http://www.breastfeeding.com/

Work and Pump
http://www.workandpump.com/

International Lactation Consultant
Association
919-861-5577
http://www.ilca.org/

Newman Breastfeeding
Clinic & Institute in the Canadian
College of Naturopathic Medicine
(CCNM)
416-498-0002
http://www.drjacknewman.com/

KellyMom
http://www.kellymom.com/

La Leche League International
800-LALECHE (525-3243)
http://www.llli.org/

World Alliance for Breastfeeding
Action (WABA)
http://www.waba.org.my/

Andi Silverman
Mamaknowsbreast.com
http://www.mamaknowsbreast.com/

Breastfeeding Café
http://www.breastfeedingcafe.com/

ProMom: Promotion of Mother's Milk, Inc.
http://www.promom.org/

National Alliance for Breastfeeding Advocacy
Barbara Heiser
http://naba-breastfeeding.org/
    index.shtml

Labor and Postpartum Doulas

DONA International
888-788-DONA (3662)
http://www.dona.org/

Association of Labor Assistants and Childbirth Educators (ALACE)
888-222-5223
http://www.alace.org/

Childbirth and Postpartum Professional Association (CAPPA)
1-888-MY-CAPPA (692-2772)
http://www.cappa.net/

Postpartum Support International
805-967-7636
http://www.postpartum.net/

National Association of Postpartum Care Services (NAPCS)
800-45-DOULA (453-6852)
http://www.napcs.org/

Exercise Resources

Baby Boot Camp
http://www.babybootcamp.com/

Itsybitsyyoga.com
http://www.itsybitsyyoga.com/

StrollerStrides
http://www.strollerstrides.com/

Beach Body
http://www.beachbody.com/

Fertility Support

Fertile Heart (Natural Options to Encourage Fertility)
http://www.fertileheart.com/

RESOLVE: The National Infertility Association
703-556-7172
http://www.resolve.org/

The Fertile Soul: Hope and Healing for Infertility
1-866-4MYFERTILITY (469-3378)
http://thefertilesoul.com/

Publications

The Compleat Mother
701-852-2822
http://www.compleatmother.com/

Fit Pregnancy **Magazine**
http://www.fitpregnancy.com/

Mindful Mama
http://www.mindfulmamamagazine
    .com/

Cookie **Magazine**
877-402-6654
http://www.cookiemag.com/

Herbs for Health **Magazine**
800-456-6018
http://www.herbsforhealth.com/

Mothering **Magazine**
Subscription Line: 800-984-8116
circulation@mothering.com
http://www.mothering.com/

Midwifery Today, Inc.
1-800-743-0974
1-541-344-7438
http://www.midwiferytoday.com/

The Bump
http://www.thebump.com/

Postpartum Depression Support

Postpartum Support International (PSI)
Postpartum Depression Helpline:
  800-944-4PPD (4773)
http://www.postpartum.net/

Depression After Delivery, Inc. (DAD)
800-944-4773
215-295-3994
http://www.depressionafterdelivery.com/

Pregnancy and Infant Loss

Share: Pregnancy & Infant Loss Support
800-821-6819
http://www.nationalshareoffice.com/

Supplies and Products

Earth Mama Angel Baby Organics
http://www.earthmamaangelbaby.com/

Birth with Love Midwifery Supplies
http://www.birthwithlove.com/

In His Hands Home Birth Supplies
http://www.inhishands.com/

Bloom
http://www.bloombaby.com/

Cascade HealthCare Products, Inc.
http://www.1cascade.com/

Herb Pharm
http://www.herb-pharm.com

Stokke
http://www.stokke.com

G Diapers
http://www.gdiapers.com/

Giggle Guide to Baby Gear
http://www.giggle.com/

Xocai Chocolate
http://www.BetterBirthbook.com/

Vaccine Information

National Vaccine Information Center
204 Mill St., Suite B1
Vienna, VA 22180
703-938-0342
http://www.909shot.com/

Videos and DVDs

Birth Day (2008), Saga Femme Productions. Starring Naoli Vinaver Lopez. Directed by Diana Paul.
http://www.amazon.com/

It's My Body, My Baby, My Birth (2007), Wisewoman Childbirth Traditions.
http://www.itsmybodymybaby mybirth.com/Home.html/

Birth into Being: The Russian Waterbirth Experence (1999), Global Maternal Child Health Association.
http://www.birthintobeing.com/

Follow Me Mum: The Key to Successful Breastfeeding (2000), Rebecca Glover.
http://www.rebeccaglover.com.au/ video.html/

Dr. Lennart Righard's Delivery Self Attachment (1992), Geddes Productions. Directed by Kittie Frantz.
http://www.geddesproduction.com/

Baby & Mom Pre Natal Yoga, Baby & Mom Post Natal Yoga
https://store.goldenbridgeyoga.com/

Birth As We Know It: The Transformative Power of Birth
http://www.birthasweknowit.com/

Orgasmic Birth (2008), Debra Pascali-Bonaro and Kris Liem.
http://www.orgasmicbirth.com/

The Business of Being Born (2007), Ricki Lake. Directed by Abby Epstein.
http://www.thebusinessofbeingborn .com/

Water Birth Resources

Waterbirth International
800-641-2229
503-673-0026
http://www.waterbirth.org/

AquaDoula
800-275-6144
425-348-6729
http://www.aquadoula.com/

Your Water Birth
509-962-8630
http://www.yourwaterbirth.com/

Web Sites

Attachment Parenting International
http://www.attachmentparenting.org/

Birthing Naturally
http://www.birthingnaturally.net/

The Family Groove
http://www.thefamilygroove.com/ index.htm/

Just Mommies
http://www.justmommies.com/

Real Savvy Moms
http://www.realsavvymoms.com/

Urban Baby
http://www.urbanbaby.com/

Kids Health
http://www.kidshealth.com/

TheNest.com
http://www.thenest.com/

Child Safety

National Crime Prevention Council (Child Safety Center)
http://www.mcgruff.org/

Safe Kids Worldwide
202-662-0600
http://www.safekids.org/

HUD Lead Listing
800-LEAD-LIST (532-3547)

National Lead Information Center
800-424-LEAD (5323)
http://www.EPA.gov/lead/

SafetyMate Inc.
800-439-8995
http://www.safetymate.com/

Other Fun Resources

Patricia Schermerhorn
Babynamer and Numerologist
415-305-7084

Spirituality for Kids
http://SFK.org/

For local resources specific to your area, please visit www .BetterBirthbook.com, where we list many amazing resources throughout the United States from midwives to prenatal yoga practitioners: all of them are friends of BornClear.

Recommended Reading

Conception

Indichova, Julia. *The Fertile Female: How the Power of Longing for a Child Can Save Your Life and Change the World.* Adell Press, 2007.

Kippley, John F. and Sheila K. Kippley. *The Art of Natural Family Planning.* Cincinnati: The Couple to Couple League, 1996.

Nofzinger, Margaret. *A Cooperative Method of Natural Birth Control.* 4th edition. Summertown, Tenn.: Book Publishing Company, 1992.

Singer, Katie. *The Garden of Fertility: A Guide to Charting Your Fertility Signals to Prevent or Achieve Pregnancy—Naturally—and to Gauge Your Reproductive Health.* New York: Avery, 2004.

Weschler, Toni. *Taking Charge of Your Fertility.* 10th edition. New York: Collins Living, 2006.

Pregnancy

Brott, Armin and Jennifer Ash. *The Expectant Father: Facts, Tips, and Advice for Dads-To-Be.* New York: Abbeville Press, 1995.

Chamberlain, David. *The Mind of Your Newborn Baby.* 3d edition. Berkeley, Calif.: North Atlantic Books, 1998.

Chopra, Deepak, David Simon and Vicki Abrams. *Magical Beginnings, Enchanted Lives.* New York: Three Rivers Press, 2005.

England, Pam and Rob Horowitz. *Birthing from Within: An Extra-Ordinary Guide to Childbirth Preparation.* Santa Barbara: Partera Press, 1998.

Gaskin, Ina May. *Ina May's Guide to Childbirth.* New York: Bantam Books, 2003.

———. *Spiritual Midwifery.* 4th edition. Summertown, Tenn.: Book Publishing Company, 2002.

Goer, Henci. *The Thinking Woman's Guide to a Better Birth.* New York: Perigee Books, 1999.

Gurmukh Kaur Khalsa. *Bountiful, Beautiful, Blissful: Experience the Natural Power of Pregnancy and Birth with Kundalini Yoga and Meditation.* New York: St. Martin's Press, 2003.

Katz Rothman, Barbara. *Encyclopedia of Childbearing.* Phoenix: Oryx Press, 1992.

Kitzinger, Sheila. *The Complete Book of Pregnancy and Childbirth.* Revised edition. New York: Knopf, 2003.

Muhlhahn, Cara. *Labor of Love: A Midwife's Memoir.* New York: Kaplan Publishing, 2008.

Odent, Michel. *The Scientification of Love.* London, Free Association Books, 1999.

Simpkin, Penny. *The Birth Partner: Everything You Need to Know to Help a Woman Through Childbirth.* 2nd edition. Boston: Harvard Common Press, 2001.

Wagner, Marsden. *Born in the USA: How a Broken Maternity System Must Be Fixed to Put Women and Children First.* Berkeley: University of California Press, 2008.

Wing, Ali. *Giggle Guide to Baby Gear.* San Francisco: Chronicle Books, 2008.

Breast-Feeding

Gaskin, Ina May. *Babies, Breastfeeding and Bonding.* Westport, Conn.: Bergin & Garvey Publishers, 1987.

La Leche League International. *The Womanly Art of Breastfeeding.* 7th revised edition. New York: Plume Books, 2004.

Renfrew, Mary, Chloe Fisher and Suzanne Arms. *Bestfeeding: Getting Breastfeeding Right for You: The Illustrated Guide.* San Francisco: Celestial Arts, 1990.

Silverman, Andi. *Mama Knows Breast: A Beginner's Guide to Breastfeeding.* Philadelphia: Quirk Books, 2007.

Sullivan, Dana and Maureen Connolly. *Unbuttoned: Women Open Up about the Pleasures, Pains, and Politics of Breastfeeding.* Boston: Harvard Common Press, 2009.

Baby and Postpartum

Hogg, Tracy with Melinda Blau. *Secrets of the Baby Whisperer: How to Calm, Connect, and Communicate with Your Baby.* New York: Ballantine Books, 2005.

Karp, Harvey. *The Happiest Kid on the Block: The New Way to Stop the Daily Battle of Wills and Raise a Secure and Well-Behaved One- to Four-Year-Old.* New York: Bantam Books, 2005.

Kitzinger, Sheila. *The Year after Childbirth: Enjoying Your Body, Your Relationships, and Yourself in Your Baby's First Year.* New York: Fireside Books, 1996.

Kunhardt, Jean, Lisa Spiegel and Sandra Kunhardt Basile. *A Mother's Circle: An Intimate Dialogue on Becoming a Mother.* 3d edition. New York: The Soho Parenting Center, 2004.

Lim, Robin. *After the Baby's Birth: A Complete Guide for Postpartum Women.* Revised edition. San Francisco: Celestial Arts, 2001.

Sears, William and Martha Sears. *The Baby Book: Everything You Need to Know about Your Baby from Birth to Age Two.* New York: Little, Brown and Company, 2003.

Parenting

Baldwin Dancy, Rahima. *You Are Your Child's First Teacher.* Revised edition. San Francisco: Celestial Arts, 2000.

Berrien Berends, Polly. *Whole Child/Whole Parent.* 4th edition. New York: HarperPerennial, 1997.

Faber, Adele and Elaine Mazlish. *How to Talk So Kids Will Listen and Listen So Kids Will Talk.* 20th edition. HarperCollins, 1999.

Kabat-Zinn, Myla and Jon Kabat-Zinn. *Everyday Blessings: The Inner Work of Mindful Parenting.* New York: Hyperion, 1998.

Kelly, Marguerite and Elia Parsons. *The Mother's Almanac.* Revised edition. New York: Broadway Books, 1975.

Kindlon, Dan and Michael Thompson. *Raising Cain: Protecting the Emotional Life of Boys.* New York: Ballantine Books, 2000.

Miller, Karen Maezen. *Momma Zen: Walking the Crooked Path of Motherhood.* Boston: Shambhala Publications, 2006.

Mogel, Wendy. *The Blessing of a Skinned Knee: Using Jewish Teachings to Raise Self-Reliant Children.* Reprint edition. New York: Scribner, 2008.

Pipher, Mary. *Reviving Ophelia: Saving the Selves of Adolescent Girls.* New York: Ballantine Books, 2002.

Small, Meredith. *Our Babies, Ourselves: How Biology and Culture Shape the Way We Parent.* New York: Anchor Books, 1999.

Self-Development

Assadi, Abdi. *Shadows on the Path.* New York: Publicide Inc., 2007.

Brach, Tara. *Radical Acceptance: Embracing Your Life with the Heart of a Buddha.* New York: Bantam Books, 2004.

Britten, Rhonda. *Fearless Living: Live without Excuses and Love without Regret.* New York: Perigee Books, 2002.

Chödrön, Pema. *The Places That Scare You: A Guide to Fearlessness in Difficult Times.* Boston: Shambhala Publications, 2007.

———. *When Things Fall Apart: Heart Advice for Difficult Times.* Boston: Shambhala Publications, 2005.

Coelho, Paulo. *The Alchemist.* New York: HarperCollins, 2006.

Chopra, Deepak. *The Seven Spiritual Laws of Success: A Pocketbook Guide to Fulfilling Your Dreams.* Abridged edition. San Rafael, Calif.: Amber-Allen Publishing, 2007.

Davis, Elizabeth. *Women's Sexual Passages: Finding Pleasure and Intimacy at Every Stage of Life.* Alameda, Calif.: Hunter House, 2000.

Davis Kasl, Charlotte. *Women, Sex, and Addiction: A Search for Love and Power.* Reprint edition. New York: HarperPerennial, 1990.

Dispenza, Joe. *Evolve Your Brain: The Science of Changing Your Mind.* Deerfield Beach, Fla.: Health Communications Inc., 2007.

Frankl, Viktor E. *Man's Search for Meaning.* 4th edition. Beacon, Mass.: Beacon Press, 2006.

Gendler, J. Ruth. *The Book of Qualities.* New York: Harper & Row, 1988.

Gladstar, Rosemary. *Herbal Healing for Women.* New York: Fireside Books, 1993.

Goddard, Neville. *The Power of Awareness.* Revised edition. Los Angeles: DeVorss & Company, 1993.

Golomb, Elan. *Trapped in the Mirror: Adult Children of Narcissists in Their Struggle for Self.* New York: William Morrow & Company, 1992.

Hay, Louise. *You Can Heal Your Life.* Carlsbad, Calif.: Hay House, 1999.

Hendrix, Harville. *Getting the Love You Want: A Guide for Couples.* Revised edition. New York: Holt Paperbacks, 2007.

Lao tzu, *Tao Te Ching.* Stephen Mitchell, trans. New York: Harper Perennial, 2006.

Luiz, Don Miguel. *The Four Agreements: A Practical Guide to Personal Freedom: A Toltec Wisdom Book.* San Rafael, Calif.: Amber-Allen Publishing, 2001.

———. *Mastery of Love: A Practical Guide to the Art of Relationship.* San Rafael, Calif.: Amber-Allen Publishing, 2002.

Miller, Alice. *The Drama of the Gifted Child: The Search for the True Self.* 3rd edition. New York: Basic Books, 2007.

Muktananda, Swami. *Where Are You Going?* 2nd edition. New Delhi: UBS Publishers Distributors, 1997.

Nhăt Hanh, Thích. *The Miracle of Mindfulness.* Mobi Ho, trans. Reprint edition. Beacon, Mass.: Beacon Press, 1999.

Northrup, Christiane. *Women's Bodies, Woman's Wisdom: Creating Physical and Emotional Health and Healing.* Revised edition. New York: Bantam Books, 2002.

Pert, Candace. *Molecules of Emotion: The Science behind Mind-Body Medicine.* New York: Simon & Schuster, 1999.

Pierakos, Eva and Judith Saly. *Creating Union: The Essence of Intimate Relationship.* 2nd edition. Charlottesville, Va.: Pathwork Press, 2002.

Shekerjian, Denise. *Uncommon Genius: How Great Ideas Are Born.* New York: Penguin Books, 1991.

Talbot, Michael. *The Holographic Universe.* New York: Harper Perennial, 1992.

Yogananda, Paramhansa. *Autobiography of a Yogi.* Reprint edition. Nevada City, Calif.: Crystal Clarity Publishers, 2003.

Index